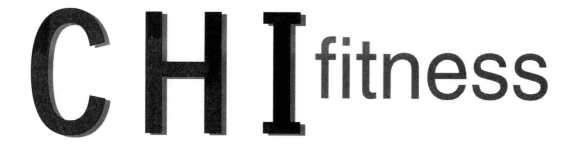

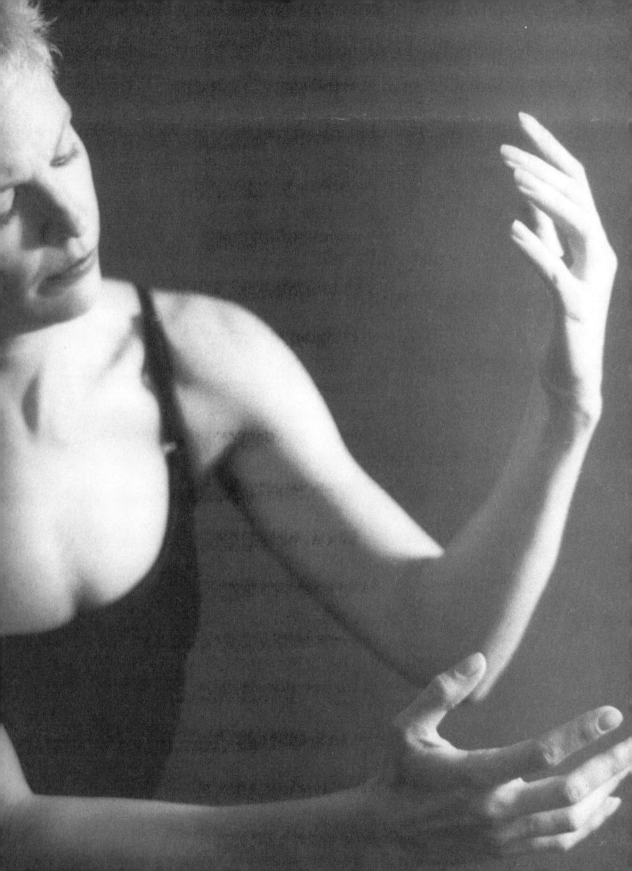

CHI fitness

A Workout for Body, Mind, and Spirit

Movements and

Meditations for

Enhancing the

Power of Your

Life Force Energy

SUE BENTON *and* DREW DENBAUM

Cliff Street Books

An Imprint of HarperCollins Publishers

The exercises and suggestions in this book are intended to supplement, not replace, the medical advice of a trained medical professional. Consult your physician before starting this exercise program. The author and publisher disclaim any liability arising directly or indirectly from the use of this book.

Some of the names and circumstances in this book have been changed or fictionalized to protect the privacy of the individuals involved.

FIRST EDITION

Designed by Mary Austin Speaker

Photographs by Andrew Brucker and MaryEllen Hendricks.

Illustrations by Yuki Hayasaki.

CHI FITNESS SM, CHI DANCE SM, *and* 🔯 SM *are service marks of Sue Benton and Drew Denbaum. All rights reserved.*

Library of Congress Cataloging-in-Publication Data is available upon request.

ISBN: 0-06-019727-7

01 02 03 04 05 ❖ / RRD 10 9 8 7 6 5 4 3 2 1

*This book is dedicated
to our parents and children,
with appreciation and love.*

Contents

Part III Chakra Power Practices

Part IV Conclusion

Introduction

Chi: Life Force Energy

Chi is the Eastern term for life force energy. It's what makes you alive. You can think of it in spiritual or medical terms, or not think of it at all, since it doesn't need your observation to function. But your conscious awareness of chi *will* affect how you live.

Most people believe that psychics or mystics are the only individuals who can perceive or channel energy. This is not true.

You don't have to be a spiritual master to acquire these simple skills. It only requires awareness and practice. Consciously connecting to your chi can put you more firmly on a path of spiritual growth and help you define healthy boundaries in your relationships.

In this book you will learn about energy and how to manage it. By performing the simple, easy-to-follow practices presented here, you will learn how to unblock and direct your energy, empowering you in every aspect of your life. You will also learn about the energy centers in your body and how to work with each one to improve your physical, emotional, and spiritual health. In the tradition of India, these energy centers are called *chakras*. Each chakra corresponds to specific physical parts of the body and also to specific areas of your life. Knowledge of your chakras will help you pinpoint the problem areas in your life and provide a basis for personal growth.

Chi is energy, and energy is power. When you allow others to control you, when you try to control others, when you can't forgive, or when chi is blocked, you are giving away your power. This ultimately causes physical illness and unhealthy relationships.

As long as you are alive, you have life force energy. *Where* you place your energy determines the quality of your life. All of us are continually bringing universal energy into our bodies, but when you give your power away, you are mismanaging your chi. In other words, you are attaching your energy to people and situations outside yourself. You are taking away the energy that runs your physical and emotional life and using it to fuel your fears. For example, if you can't forgive someone, you are sending your chi back into the past to keep your hurt or anger alive. It takes energy to stay mad.

When your energy is blocked, that is also due to fear. For instance, if you repress your sexual feelings, you will restrict the flow of chi through your sexual organs, creating an energy block in that part of your body. The end result of giving away or blocking your chi is that you don't have as much energy to create the life you want and maintain a healthy body.

Love empowers and fear disempowers you. Throughout this book, we will discuss in detail how fear and love affect your life force energy in different ways. Controlling behavior, for instance, is fear-based. When you are attempting to control another person, you have an investment in how he behaves. If he doesn't behave the way you want, you have to expend even more power to enforce your control. When you are in a position of leadership or parenting, instead of doing it in a fear-based way, you can *guide* others by inspiring or teaching them without relinquishing your power or usurping theirs. You might be thinking, "I have to control my children, don't I?" It's certainly important to set limits for our children. It's important to set boundaries in any relationship. But it's also clear that setting limits can either empower or disempower. You can protect others by helping them learn how to take care of themselves, for example, or you can simply restrict their behavior in a way that feels imprisoning. Respecting someone else's individuality and capacity for growth is empowering and rooted in love.

Relinquishing your power can happen both instantaneously and over time. You can relinquish it to a parent, to a set of beliefs about yourself, or to old wounds over the course of your entire life. On the other hand, you can surrender your chi in a second to a stranger on the street who is rude to you. Chi Fitness will enable you to take your power back in any situation, whether it is happening in the present or stems from the past.

Love always empowers both you and those you love. When you are loving someone, you are sending him positive energy. That helps him and also empowers you. However, what you experience as love could be rooted in fear. For example, someone who needs to dominate another person may think he is doing so out of love, but such behavior is actually fear-based. Loving someone is wanting for her what she wants for herself—not only what *you* want for her. If you are trying to control someone's behavior, that's not really love; that's attachment through fear.

Movement as Metaphor

The body stores all of your experience, all of your thoughts and feelings. Traumas and blocks are evident in the way you move, since *movement is a metaphor for life.* When the body is tight, chi cannot flow. In this book we teach you how to use the body and chi as the means to promote spiritual growth and healing.

We've all been in situations in which we react with fear. Our breathing becomes very fast and shallow. In that moment it's almost impossible to think clearly. Most of us know that if you take deep breaths, you automatically start to calm down so that you can begin to think coherently. This is the approach we are using when we are managing our chi. We use specific techniques to direct the flow of energy through our bodies, so that we can be "in our power" in any given moment. As you discover your chi and become aware of the chakra system, you will *feel* when you are restricting the flow of energy in your body. This starts a healing process that begins energetically with awareness and management of your chi, then affects the body and the mind.

When you have relinquished your chi, you may feel an emotional "charge" such as upset, anger, or jealousy, or you may feel physically drained of energy, even depressed. Usually when we are in a situation that saps our energy, we are caught off-guard and are not able to identify exactly what's going on. Once you have learned what it feels like to be in your power, you will immediately recognize when you have relinquished your chi. This is something you will actually feel in your body. You may feel physically off-balance. You may feel pain or pressure in a particular area of your body. The physical sensation will be very clear to you and signal you to take your chi back instantly. This will help you think more clearly and respond better to the situation.

This book presents Power Practices that will teach you to feel and direct your chi and free up the flow of energy in the areas of your body corresponding to each of your chakras. Included in each exercise are metaphors connecting the physical movement to a specific aspect of your life.

These Power Practices also reveal where you give your power away—to some person or experience that hurt you now or in the past, or to an erroneous belief system that no longer serves you. You will learn how to *reclaim your chi* and embody authentic power—not power over others, but true, internal power.

Simple guided meditations and visualizations are placed throughout the book to unblock your energy centers and assist you in every aspect of your life, such as decision making, releasing fear, forgiving, and deepening your relationships and self-esteem. Each level of exercise also includes an affirmation to use as the basis of brief, centering meditations throughout the day.

How to Use This Book

Chi Fitness takes you step-by-step through a process of managing your life force energy. First, there are Basic Power Practices that increase your facility to feel your energy, consciously manage it, and remain empowered in any circumstance. Once you master the Basic Power Practices, you can progress in your energy work by using the Chakra Power Practices, which apply these basic exercises to specific chakras. Each chakra correlates to different aspects of your life. The Chakra Power Practices are designed to free up the flow of energy in all of your energy centers. This process leads to self-discovery and an opportunity to heal old wounds and stay in your power. The Chakra Power Practices are presented at various levels, corresponding to physical exertion. The short practices can be done anywhere, at any time.

When you are using the Basic Power Practices for managing your chi, you will go through four steps:

1. Feel the physical sensation of your chi.

2. Realize that you are blocking your energy or giving your power away.

3. Use a Basic Power Practice. You can use one of these practices the moment you relinquish your chi or perform these techniques at your leisure during quiet time or meditation.

4. Utilize the Four Questions for Healing and "self-talk" to explore why you behave in certain situations the way you do. For example, if you are constantly losing your power in similar situations and want to look deeper, this is a method to help you begin a healing process.

The Four Questions utilize all of the Basic Power Practices along with self-talk to help you discover the roots of your behavior so that you can be in your power in any circumstance. Self-talk encourages you to nurture yourself as you would a beloved child or dear friend.

When you experience a charge in your emotions (such as anger, anxiety, or resentment) indicating that you have given away your chi, you can immediately use a Basic Power Practice. Say you are in a situation with your sister. She has just made you very angry. You perceive that you are giving away your chi. In that moment, you use one of the Basic Power Practices to call back your energy. When you get home, you are still annoyed. Since you and your sister have many of these episodes, you want to explore the situation. You take some quiet time for yourself and do a longer version of the Basic Practice. You may then choose to ask yourself the Four Questions for Healing, followed by self-talk. Using these techniques will allow you to practice taking your chi back from your sister and discover the root cause of your anger so you can let it go once and for all. The Basic Power Practices also provide you with the means to understand the lessons that incidents like this carry.

Chakra Power Practices come into play once you have the facility to feel exactly where in your body you are losing your chi. As with the Basic Power Practices, there is a progression of steps to follow:

1. Feel the physical sensation of your chi.

2. Realize that you are blocking your energy or giving your power away.

3. Associate that restriction or power loss with a particular energy center in your body and connect that energy center with an aspect of your life.

4. Use a Chakra Power Practice. You can use a short practice in the moment and later do the movement exercise and meditations for that energy center to unblock and direct your chi.

5. Use the Four Questions for Healing and self-talk.

For example, if someone ridicules something you've said, it's natural to feel upset. If you realize that your emotional reaction means that you have relinquished your energy, you have already accomplished the first two steps of both Basic and Chakra Power Practices. In Step 3 of this example, you may notice that you feel off-balance or even hurt in the area of your solar plexus. Since this is the location of the third chakra, it would indicate that the criticism is affecting your self-esteem. Another person in the same situation might be affected in the second chakra (the lower abdominal area), indicating that the issue is about a power struggle. In Step 4, you can use a Short Practice while the incident is occurring and later refer to the exercises and meditations for the appropriate chakra. These steps will assist you in keeping your chi flowing through your body. In Step 5, you can explore the insights you receive by using the Four Questions for Healing and self-talk.

Performing these practices allows you to regain your power in the particular situation that upset you. You will then be able to deal with the circumstance from a powerful, loving perspective rather than from a position of disempowerment and fear. These practices also help you discover whether the disturbance is rooted in an old wound or behavior pattern, or relates to a self-esteem problem that needs to be healed.

There are five Basic Power Practices concerned directly with managing your chi. In the Chakra Power Practices, there are four levels of movement for each chakra so you can choose which level of exercise you want to do. One day you may feel quite vigorous and choose to do the Level 3 exercise for a particular chakra. If you've had a bad night's sleep, you might choose to do Level 1 or the Short Practice. The Short Practice is the simplest and most subtle form, from a physical standpoint. The Level 1 exercise is an easy movement to perform. Levels 2 and 3 are increasingly physically demanding. One level of exercise is not better than another when it comes to moving and unblocking energy. The difference lies only in the amount of physical exertion required to do each level.

When you exercise your physical body, your muscles become more responsive to your will. It is the same with your energy system. The more you exercise and practice commanding your chi, the easier it will be to remain empowered. This is the meaning of the name *Chi Fitness*. Just as physical exercise makes your body fit, Chi Fitness helps you put your life force energy under your conscious control.

At each level of exercise, there is a movement metaphor to connect your physical action to your energetic, emotional, and psychological state of being. There is also an affirmation for each level of practice to help you make this connection. Choose the practice you want to perform according to how you feel.

The meditations in this book are not meant to be memorized. Simply incorporate their essence into your own Meditation Practice. If you do not meditate, use these thoughts and ideas in any quiet, solitary time you set aside for yourself. It is essential for your overall well-being to have solitude, even if it's only for fifteen minutes a day. You need time alone to attain a sense of mastery over your life and to "refuel." Otherwise, your energy will be scattered over all the events and people you come into contact with throughout your day. If you take the time to ground yourself through Power Practices and meditation, you will find that it seems you have more than enough time to do what you need to do. You will have empowered yourself to approach your daily tasks from a foundation of peace, instead of running around with your chi scattered, "putting out fires" all day.

Having read this far, you have already learned the basis of Chi Fitness. The rest of the book will guide you through practices that empower you to feel and function better every day of your life.

PART I

Discovering Your Chi

Chi is the life force energy that makes you a living being. It is the central, animating element of your overall energy system. Every living thing has chi. Inanimate objects also have energy, but not conscious awareness. According to ancient Eastern philosophies (Jainism, for example), energy is differentiated into *sentient* and *insentient*. Sentient energy is conscious awareness (*atma*). Insentient energy manifests itself in either tangible or intangible forms: unconscious matter or movement, rest, space, and time. Even though these beliefs are thousands of years old, they presage many aspects of modern physics. Whatever system of thought you follow, as a sentient being you can learn to manage your chi to realize your highest potential.

As we touched on in the Introduction, many people think that only psychics can see and direct energy.

Authentic psychics and mystics have a natural gift for using their intuition and channeling chi. Think of natural athletes. Their ability to move their bodies effectively is an inborn talent. This doesn't mean that those of us who are not as gifted cannot learn to be excellent athletes, too. It is the same with our facility to manage our life force energy. We all possess an innate ability to do this, but it requires awareness and practice to master.

The following chapters present specific exercises that make up Step 1, feeling your chi. You might know what chi is intellectually, but knowing what it is doesn't necessarily give you an awareness of what it feels like. What we are trying to do in this book is give you the *physical experience* of your chi so that when you give it away, you will distinctly feel its loss and be able to draw it back.

These practices will help you feel and see both your own chi and the life force energy of those around you. You will physically experience energy being moved by your thoughts and intentions.

Chapter 1

FEELING AND SEEING YOUR CHI

Remember high school science class? We learned that everything in the world is made up of atoms. Our bodies, the trees, the chair that you are sitting on are all made of the same stuff, organized in different patterns. An atom is made up of particles in its center (protons and neutrons); particles revolving around its center (electrons); and the energy in between, which keeps the electrons in orbit and prevents the nucleus from flying apart. The atom is 99.9 percent energy, and at the atomic level *we* are 99.9 percent energy.

Chi is your life force energy. It is already within you. There is no trick to feeling it or seeing it. It only requires attention and practice to do so. The following exercises illustrate ways to experience chi physically.

Chi Ball Exercise

1. Stand with your feet about hip distance apart. Straighten the spine by lifting up through the crown of the head and gently pressing down through the tailbone. Notice that when you straighten the spine, you automatically take a deep breath as you create more space in your body. All the joints should be soft and relaxed: knees, hips, elbows, shoulders, and ankles.

2. Bend the knees slightly over the toes.

3. Draw your hands up to waist level with the palms facing each other.

Relax your fingers and bring your awareness to the palms of your hands. Imagine that you are holding a ball of energy.

Keep in mind that it is important to maintain a state of relaxation. This is not a test. It's an exploration. It should be fun. After a moment or two, you will feel a tingling sensation, heat, or perhaps a vibration between the palms of your hands.

If you are not perceiving any of these sensations, try moving the palms of your hands toward each other, then away from each other, in a gentle, pulsing motion. Soon you will begin to sense the chi between your hands. Visualize it as a ball of energy.

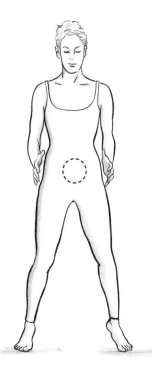

As you become increasingly aware of this chi ball, look at the area around your hands. If you place your hands over a darker surface, you may begin to see an outline of energy. Relax your gaze; don't use a hard stare. Sometimes, you can see what looks like white smoke between the fingers of both hands. Some people can even see colors. These are aspects of your aura.

The aura is the energy field that surrounds all matter. If something has an atomic structure, it will have an aura. If it is alive, the auric field will be more intense. The size and shape of your aura, as well as the colors and clarity of the colors, signify different things about your physical, emotional, psychological, and spiritual well-being.

As you're learning to see the aura, it's important to remember not to stare because what looks like an aura around an individual could be an optical illusion. When you stare fixedly at an object, your eye muscles become fatigued. The resulting shift in focus can cause you to see an after-image that looks like an aura. Relaxing your gaze will help you see the energy of another person.

Here are some additional ways to perceive energy:

Try doing the Chi Ball Exercise in front of a full-length mirror. If you wear darker clothing, this exercise will be easier. As you sense the energy between your hands, look in the mirror. You may see the ball of energy in the mirror as well as between and around your hands.

Have a friend stand in front of a blank wall and look at him. Soft focus your eyes and try to see the energy surrounding him. *Don't discount what you see.* Energy is a palpable experience, and seeing it is fully within your power.

As you look at your friend, you may see just an outline around him, white light, or colors. Keep in mind that you may be the kind of person who *feels* energy more readily than seeing it. On the other hand, you may have the experience of seeing energy, but not specific colors. Some people never see colors. Other people always do. Others see colors sometimes. It depends on what you are sensitive to. Practice will sharpen your skill, so keep trying. (Remember to soft focus your eyes and *relax*.) Certain people learn better visually, some aurally, and others somatically. One way is not better than the other. Whatever way you sense chi is the perfect way for you.

Colors in an energy field close to the body reflect your physical health. Colors perceived farther away from the body have to do with emotional and spiritual states. There are many different ways to interpret the meaning of particular colors. It is widely believed that the clarity and vibrancy of color are indications of the energy's intensity. Dull or washed-out color can indicate energy imbalances or depletion. Keep in mind that just as modern physics recognizes the effect that any observer has on an experiment, your own state of being will undoubtedly affect your perception of anyone else's aura. In addition, these colors can change repeatedly, indicating variations in a person's physical, emotional, or spiritual state of being. Ask questions of the people you are studying to gain insights about their state of being and trust your intuition.

When you have an extra moment, practice the Chi Ball Exercise to enhance your awareness of chi. As you go through your day, try to see the energy of other people. Practicing your newfound awareness of chi increases your skill at sensing energy.

Chapter 2

ENERGY FOLLOWS INTENTION

There are two basic emotions: love and fear. Love is joy, acceptance, and the entire spectrum of positive emotions. When we are loving someone, we are sending him a beam or vibration of love and light. This assists the other person because he is receiving positive energy, and, at the same time, it empowers *you*. When you are angry at someone, you are disempowering yourself by giving away your chi, while the other person is receiving the vibration of your negative energy.

Reading this might give you the idea

that because anger is disempowering you should not get angry. This is not so. It is very important to express your positive *and* negative emotions, including anger, honestly. We are spiritual beings having a human adventure. Part of the joy of being human is experiencing our true feelings. When you are angry, allow yourself to feel it thoroughly. The trap is getting *stuck* in angry emotions. You continue to relinquish your chi when you hold on to your anger by acting out your rage or ruminating over the incident that made you mad. If an emotion is fear-based, you can reclaim your chi by using a Power Practice and the Four Questions for Healing to discover what is motivating your reaction.

If someone is angry and sends you negative thoughts, you don't have to be influenced by them. You won't be affected if you don't participate by getting angry in return or feeling upset. If you are in your power, that negative energy won't disturb you.

Fear is the root of all our negative emotions. Think about it. When you are angry, you are actually afraid. When you are judging someone, you are afraid. When you are jealous or envious, that is fear, too. Any emotion that is not rooted in love is based in fear. If you look behind any negative emotion, you will see this. Take boredom, for example. If you look underneath the emotion of boredom, you'll probably find restlessness. Under the restlessness could very well be frustration. Why are you frustrated? Perhaps there are things you really want to do but are afraid to try. The same reasoning could be applied to any negative emotion you are feeling.

Most people feel that hate is the opposite of love. Underlying hate is fear. To recognize this, you can apply the same process we went through in the last paragraph: You hate someone. Why? Go underneath your hatred. Maybe you'll find jealousy. Explore its cause. Perhaps you see this person as having more success than you. Does that bother you? If you subconsciously think you'll never be as successful, it probably makes you afraid. The scenario could also go this way: Why do you hate a certain individual? You hate the way he acts because you think he is arrogant. Why does his arrogance bother you? Because it seems that he thinks you're worthless. Why should that upset you? Perhaps deep down you think you *are* worthless and this frightens you. Apply this process to any negative emotion, and at its source, you will find fear.

As you explore the root of your feelings and how they relate to the flow of energy in yourself and your relationships, what if you have emotions toward certain people in your life that don't feel like either love or fear? Take your relationship with your employer, as an example. You may not love or even like your boss, but your interaction with him will be either based in fear or rooted in love. If you're anticipating his negative judgment, your relationship with him is colored by a fear-based expectation. On the other hand, even if you don't like your boss, your relationship with him can be based in love. You can perform your job without relinquishing your power to anxious anticipation of what's going to happen next. You can be present in the moment, respecting your own position and that of your boss, without feeling threatened.

When we make a decision, it is based on either love or fear. If we choose from a place of fear, the consequences of that decision will reflect fear. When we make a love-based decision, the result reflects that loving intention. Many embrace the belief that each soul incarnates on Earth to learn lessons in order to grow toward a state of perfection. Therefore, your soul creates the experiences you need for personal growth. For example, if you are living a life based in fear, your soul will create experiences that are frightening so that you can have the opportunity to overcome your fear. This, in turn, will eventually teach you that fear doesn't work as a way to live your life in alignment with your soul. These issues are discussed in greater detail in Chapter 21, "Creating Your Reality."

When you look at life from this point of view, you may wonder why awful things happen to good people. It's hard not to question the principle of creating your own reality in this context. Embracing this belief, however, will enable you to see that when something horrible happens, on some level a person's soul grows from every experience. Many people believe that past lives affect their present situation as well. In any event, it's a matter of faith to accept that whatever you experience on Earth is for the purpose of your soul's growth, however terrible or "unjustified" it may seem.

It's essential not to blame yourself for negative experiences. Whether it is part of "God's plan" or is simply necessary for the growth of your soul, *blame* has no positive role in the equation. This is why so many philosophies teach *equanimity* as the key to happiness, as is wonderfully expressed by the Serenity Prayer: "God grant me the serenity to accept the things I cannot change, the strength to change the things I can, and the wisdom to know the difference."

Accepting what happens in your life, however, doesn't mean giving in to heartache or failure. Chi Fitness is all about your empowerment and growth—spiritually, emotionally, and physically.

Your thoughts and intentions actually *move* and *direct* your chi. You create your reality with your thoughts and intentions. If there are people in your past you cannot forgive, you are sending your energy back into the past every time you think about them. You are using your energy to maintain your anger. Since anger is fear, fear is your intention, whether you realize it or not. In other words, the thoughts and feelings you experience in these moments grow out of your fear.

When you worry about what *might* happen, you are sending your energy forward to negative probabilities of what may occur in your future. Again, your intention is rooted in fear.

When we are not angry about the past or anxious about the future, our power is not spread out over a period of time. Our chi is concentrated in the present moment. We are in our power and are able to create our reality with love and faith.

The following exercises demonstrate that your thoughts and intentions direct your energy.

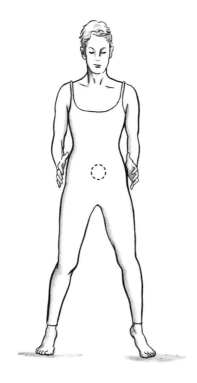

Tennis Ball Exercise

1. Stand with your feet about hip distance apart. Straighten the spine by lifting up through the crown of the head and pushing down through the tailbone. As in the Chi Ball Exercise, all the joints are soft and relaxed, with the knees slightly bent over the toes.

2. Lift the palms of your hands, facing them together about waist high. Feel the energy ball, about the size of a tennis ball, between your hands. Stay with this perception until the sensation feels strong.

3. Without moving your hands, use the intention of your mind to make the tennis ball bounce from your left hand to your right hand and back again. You will actually feel as though the tennis ball is lobbing back and forth between your hands. Play with this sensation by making the ball go

faster. Now slow the tennis ball down. This exercise powerfully illustrates that your intention is in charge of the movement of your chi.

Snowball Exercise

1. Stand with your feet about hip distance apart. Straighten the spine by lifting up through the crown of the head and pushing down through the tailbone. As in the preceding exercises, all the joints are soft and relaxed, and the knees are slightly bent over the toes.

2. Lift the palms of your hands, facing them together about waist high. Feel the energy between the hands.

3. Draw the hands together just as if you were packing snow into the size of a Ping-Pong ball. Keep pressing the hands together in this motion, packing the "snow" into a compact ball. Feel the density of the energy as you do this exercise.

4. Pull your hands farther apart to about the size of a baseball. Use the same hand motions as before. Be aware of how dense and solid your chi feels between your hands while performing this exercise.

5. Move the hands even farther apart and make a snowball the size of a basketball, staying aware of how solid your energy feels when this is your intention.

Disk Exercise

1. Stand with your feet about hip distance apart. Straighten the spine by lifting up through the crown of the head and pushing down through the tailbone. As in the preceding exercises, all the joints are soft and relaxed, and the knees are slightly bent over the toes.

2. Pretend that you are holding between your hands a disk about the size and shape of a Frisbee. Without moving your hands, using just your intention, make this disk turn in your hands to the left. Feel the disk turning between your hands from the right hand to the left.

3. Try making the rotation of the disk slow down. Then make it go faster. Now change the direction of the disk so that it circles from left to right.

If you have trouble doing these exercises because you can't feel your chi yet, make sure that you are relaxed and breathing normally, with all of your joints soft and your spine straight. Hands should be in a firm yet relaxed pose. Place your awareness between the palms of the hands. If you still don't perceive anything, pulse your hands closer, then farther apart (moving them only about an inch, in and out). Continue this pulsing motion. If you still don't perceive anything, you probably just need to ease up and let go of any anxiety about this. Eventually you *will* feel your energy. Just keep trying.

Just as your intention controls the movement of the tennis ball, the size and density of the snowball, and the rotation of the disk, so it is in your life. Your intention creates your reality. The result of every decision you make is colored by the energy of the intention with which you have rendered it.

Our intentions form on both conscious and unconscious levels. A conscious intention to manifest love can be undermined by an unconscious motivation that is rooted in fear. Chi Fitness practices will work on both levels, since movement is a metaphor for life, and the flow of energy through your body will break through physical, emotional, and energetic blocks. You don't need to be aware of how or why Chi Fitness works to feel better as a result of these practices, but your awareness and understanding will increase naturally as you learn to take charge of your chi.

Perhaps you have always been told that "there is not enough to go around": not enough money, not enough love. If this is your core belief, however unconscious, the intentions that you send out will be colored by a sense of lack. Therefore, the outward attributes of your life will mirror that basic sensibility. When you learn to take charge of your chi and use your body to allow your chi to flow, you will be able to change any root ideas that don't serve you. Our core beliefs inform our thoughts and our thoughts give birth to our intentions. Often we are not aware of our true core beliefs and we create conditions in our lives that we really do not want. Becoming aware of your chi, managing it, and using the body to allow its free flow are ways Chi Fitness enables you to change your undesirable root convictions to thoughts that help you create the life you desire.

It's common for people to think it is appropriate to base a course of action on fear: "I can't quit this job I hate because I'm afraid I'll starve." "I can't leave my abusive boyfriend because I'm scared to be alone." When a decision is fear-based, the outcome is self-defeating because it puts you on a path that is not fulfilling. In the first example, the person stays in a job out of fear. What is the result? He continues to live an existence he can't stand. He may be eating, but he's also being eaten up inside. Fear keeps you stuck in the same unhappy situation.

In the second example, the woman stays in an abusive relationship, not recognizing the choices she has to improve her life because of her terror. If she could make a decision based on love, she would never allow herself to be abused. Even if she loved her abuser, she would recognize that the relationship is destructive to both of them. Making a loved-based choice would give her the opportunity to find a relationship that would empower her.

This is not to say that you should act without an awareness of consequences. It just means you must be careful to recognize your true motivation. Is it fear or love? If you choose with the intention of love, the result will ultimately reflect that love and empower you.

A Personal Note

Soon after I was divorced, I decided to get a second graduate degree, one that was highly marketable. My first love was dance and movement, but I had two children to support and was afraid to strike out on my own. Right before I was to start school, I got a very attractive offer to head the mind-body fitness department of a new spa. This, I thought, would be perfect. I would have job security and I could do the work I loved. I negotiated a good salary. I chose to take this job because I was afraid to do what I really wanted to do: open my own studio. So here I was, depending on somebody else to do for me what I was too afraid to do for myself. I chose out of fear, thinking that this choice would produce security for me and my children.

Since the intention of a choice affects its consequences, the entire job blew up in my face. I was then faced with another decision. I could stay in the job at half-salary, which was financially impossible for me, or I could start my own business. I was terrified and upset by this turn of events.

Without realizing at the time what I was doing, I took my power back by using "self-talk," which went something like this: "I don't enjoy working there. If I take half-salary, I'll have to get another job and I'll be running back and forth like a lunatic. I won't be able to spend much time with my kids. Is it really worth it? Absolutely not." I also told myself, "Hey, you're not stupid, and you're good at what you do. If it doesn't work out, you'll figure out something else." I went back the next day and, much to my employer's surprise, announced that I'd stay for another month at full salary, then leave. Afterward, I opened Chi Fitness—a decision made from love and not fear.

Jeffrey's experience

It took Jeffrey until he was an adult to understand the fear-based behavior that afflicted him as a child. With the hindsight of an adult and a knowledge that one's core beliefs are based in either fear or love, Jeffrey can look at his past experience and understand its fear-based roots.

As a five-year-old, Jeffrey knew how it felt to have his energy blocked by a core belief, even though he didn't realize it at the time. At home and at school, he was precocious, excelling intellectually beyond the expectations of his age level. Jeffrey's parents praised and encouraged him. He seemed to be developing well—except in one area: he was so shy that he could hardly speak. Thoughts rushed into his mind, but he found it nearly impossible to express himself in public. He could actually feel the words welling up and sticking in his throat, then had to endure the taunts of his classmates while doing his best to keep up a brave front. Jeffrey's teachers and parents were always reassuring, but he could tell they were dismayed. He was taken to child psychologists, but the problem persisted.

Jeffrey now realizes that his core belief system was grounded in fear. Even though his parents were almost always outwardly supportive and loving, his experience of home life was like a roller coaster ride, with highs of affection and happiness swerving and falling at a moment's notice into lows of acrimony and tears. He always felt that, at any moment, the rug could be pulled out from under him, and any transgression could be linked to any offense he'd ever committed. This fear permeated his psyche. Like most children, he subconsciously blamed himself for what went wrong, undermining his self-esteem and crippling his ability to "speak his truth."

Happily, Jeffrey found ways to express himself creatively that circumnavigated these psychological and emotional blocks, starting in childhood and continuing through adulthood, but it wasn't until he recently explored them on an energetic level that he really began to feel at peace about what went on and understand how to reclaim his chi in these areas of his life. Jeffrey's shyness and speech impediment were a symptom of fear that everything could fall apart at a moment's notice. He was afraid that his words could cause an explosive situation. Therefore, it was difficult for him to speak. Even after he overcame his shyness, this particular fear-based core belief exhibited itself in other ways until he learned how to reclaim his chi and explore the causes of his energy block.

Chapter 3

TOTAL BODY CHI

In Eastern medicine, healers use pathways of chi called *energy meridians*. These meridians run through the body distributing life force energy to the physical being. The body also contains seven energy centers called *chakras* that are located within the core of the body. For most people, it is generally easiest to feel chi in the hands. Now we will work to enhance your perception of chi throughout your body.

Total Body Chi

1. Sit in a comfortable position with your spine straight and your feet flat on the floor.

2. Place the hands waist high, palms facing each other. Feel the energy between your hands and take deep relaxing breaths. Continue feeling the chi between your hands as you close your eyes.

3. Place your hands, palms up, resting on your knees, feeling the energy in the palms of your hands.

4. Trace the energy from your hands up your arms, then down through your body all the way through the soles of your feet. Don't feel that you have to identify specific energy pathways. Just get a sense of the chi flowing through your entire physique.

5. Feel the general vibration of your life force energy throughout your whole body, from the top of your head out through your fingers through the soles of your feet. This is a wonderful way to quiet your mind when you begin a meditation. Just relax into the pleasant tingling of your chi.

Total Body Chi and Weight Loss

Often an individual will overeat, not because she is hungry, but because she has fear-based emotions. When a person is fearful, she is giving away her chi. Her energy is scattered elsewhere when she feels these uncomfortable feelings and, mistakenly, thinks she needs to eat, unaware of whether she is actually hungry or full. She continues to eat because she is not interpreting the signals of her body correctly.

A way to stop this habit of overeating is to feel your total body chi periodically throughout the day. When you are feeling your chi, make sure that you are using your intention to distribute it all over your body: up through your head, out your arms, down your spine and through the soles of your feet. Remember, don't do this only when you feel hungry. Take the time to do it a number of times each day. Not only will it get you more in touch with your chi and your body, but it will be a minimeditation that will ground and calm you.

Please note: Extreme overeating has many psychological and metabolic causes. This practice is not meant to be a substitute for medical or therapeutic support. It can, however, get anyone more in touch with messages the body is sending.

Other People's Chi

We've all had the experience of feeling a kinship with someone we just met. It's also common to feel immediately repelled when meeting someone for the first time, but be careful about labeling another person's chi as "negative." When you feel uncomfortable being with another person and you don't quite know why, it is because you are picking up on an energetic cue. What is known as "chemistry" between two people does not apply only to lovers, but to friends, families, and coworkers as well. There are some people you just don't feel attracted to and you can sense this on an energetic level, even though you can't quite put your feelings into words. It is important to acknowledge your initial perceptions of incompatibility, but it is also important not to judge someone, especially on the basis of a first impression. Instinctive repulsion can prove to be well-founded, but there are also times when an initial aversion can change to compassion and even attraction when we get to know someone on a more intimate level.

Have you ever walked into a room where two people are behaving normally, but—even though you didn't witness or hear any conflict between them—you *know* that they've had an argument? Think of all the times you have known, without being told, that someone dear to you is upset. Maybe you see him at work every day. He is acting the same as always—the same greetings to others, the same banter. No one else notices that he's upset, but you do. Why? Without consciously realizing it, you read his energy every day. His energy is so familiar to you that you know when it's "off," no matter how he's behaving.

The following exercises practice consciously perceiving other people's chi.

Exercise 1

1. Get a partner to do this exercise with you. You are the giver and he is the receiver.

2. Have the receiver stand about two feet away from you. Both of you should stand with your feet about hip distance apart. Straighten the spine by lifting up through the crown of the head and pushing down through the tailbone. As in the preceding exercises, all joints should be soft and relaxed, with knees slightly bent over the toes.

3. The receiver stands in this position with hands relaxed and at his sides. You face the receiver and feel a ball of energy between the palms of your hands. Make it about the size of a volleyball. Stay in this position until you have a strong sense of the energy between your hands.

4. Push the chi ball to the receiver so that he can get the experience of directly feeling your energy. It takes *relaxed* awareness to sense the chi.

5. Do this several times until the receiver physically feels your energy. Then switch roles so that you become the receiver.

If you find that you can feel your own chi but not your partner's, take a deep breath, relax, and try again. Receiving the chi ball often does not feel like catching a real ball. Many people describe the other person's energy as "washing over" their bodies. Imagine someone throwing a water balloon at you in slow motion. It "breaks" on contact and the other person's energy feels like the "water" cascading over your body.

Exercise 2

1. Have your partner lie down on the floor with his spine straight in a relaxed position, eyes closed. Make sure he is taking deep, full, long breaths.

2. Sit next to him and place your hands on either side of your partner's calf muscle, keeping a distance of about three inches between your hands and your partner's leg. Feel the energy ball between the palms of your hands passing through his calf. Ask your partner what he feels.

3. Do the Tennis Ball Exercise. Send the energy from one palm to the other through your partner's calf muscle. Ask him what he feels.

4. Try the Snowball Exercise, compacting the energy between the palms of your hands, with your partner's leg in between.

5. Do the Rotating Disk Exercise, circling the energy through the calf muscle of your partner.

After you do this for a while, see whether your partner can identify which exercise you are doing by sensing your energy in his leg. Switch places and let your partner do the exercises as you try to identify each one.

Exercise 3

1. You sit comfortably in a chair with your spine straight and your feet flat on the floor. Close your eyes and get a sense of your total body chi.

2. Your partner chooses where to move in the room, *silently*. He can move away from you, toward you, behind you, or to your right or left.

3. Every twenty seconds or so, you verbally announce where your partner is in the room by homing in on his energy.

You will find that everybody has a distinct energy signature you can identify with practice and awareness. You can do Exercise 3 with several of your friends. Have one person close his eyes, and have the other participants take turns entering the room. See how accurately he can perceive and identify each person's chi signature. With practice, a friend's energy will be as familiar to you as his voice on the phone.

We all possess a natural perception of the energy around us. To draw the language of energy into our consciousness, we can enhance our natural perception of chi by practicing these exercises, just as we practice honing any skill. We can also practice by noticing our reactions to people, places, and situations by physically perceiving the chi around us. When you walk into a store or the place where you work, ask yourself how you feel about the energy there. The energy of a store can depend on many variables, such as the people who work there, the intentions of the people who founded it, and what the business sells. If the people who founded the store and the people who work there have a service mentality and enjoy their jobs, the chi in that store will be very different from that in a place where its employees are pressured to make a sale at any cost. What the store sells is also very important. The energy you would find in a store that sells baby furniture is going to be very different from the chi in a gun store. The way the chi flows through a building is also significant. There is an Eastern art called *Feng Shui* that focuses on architecture and the placement of objects to optimize the flow of energy in a room or structure.

Our world and all of the beings that inhabit it are 99.9 percent energy. The perception of chi is the first step in learning to manage the energy that empowers you and your life.

PART II

Basic Power Practices

As stated in the Introduction, there are four steps to managing your chi in your everyday life.

Step 1: Awareness of your chi. This means that you are conscious of it and have the physical experience of feeling your energy. You can practice this step simply by feeling the energy between the palms of your hands, moving it with your intention, and progressing to feeling it throughout your entire body. (These practices are presented in Part I.)

Step 2: Realizing when your energy is blocked or when you are giving your power away. To experience this sensation you must practice and memorize how you feel when you are in your power, and contrast this with how you feel when you are giving your power away. You will learn to do this by using one of the Basic Power Practices, Power in Present Time. From this exercise, you will become more and more familiar with your chi and you will be able to recognize when you are giving your power away. It will be a physical experience, as easily recognizable as a shot in the arm.

Step 3: Taking your power back the moment you feel yourself losing it, using any of the Basic Power Practices.

Step 4: Asking yourself the Four Questions for Healing and using self-talk.

There are five Basic Power Practices presented in Part II. They are:

1. Breath
2. Power in Present Time and its addendum, Experiencing Power Loss
3. Reclaiming Your Chi
4. Letting Go of Fear
5. Spiritual Perspective

Part II ends with a presentation of the Four Questions for Healing and self-talk, along with practices that assist your spiritual growth and empowerment.

Chapter 4

BREATH

One of our favorite quotes is from Dr. Moshe Feldenkrais, a pioneer of body-based therapy. He said, "You can't change the body without changing the mind, and you can't change the mind without changing the body." The body is the manifestation of all our experience. It is the physical embodiment of our inner life, as well as our past.

Breath is the bridge between the body and the mind.

Breathing is both a voluntary and an involuntary function. When we are overcome by fear, our breathing automatically becomes shallow and fast. The body then starts to mobilize its muscles for action, fight or flight. The breath acts as a bridge because, in the moment of your fear, your emotions first create fast, shallow breathing, which in turn signals the body to react. If you are able to breathe deeply and fully, your body's reaction will be more under your control, and that control is a key to your empowerment.

The primal "fight or flight" response mobilizes your body's resources to deal with a dangerous situation. When you react with fear, you give away a great deal of your energy to the outside source of danger. This sends your body into the fight or flight mode. Biologically, the sympathetic branch of your autonomic nervous system comes into play, releasing adrenaline into the bloodstream and stimulating the muscles to fight or flee. Any fear-based response goes through the same process, whether it is physical or emotional. The amount of chi you lose depends upon the intensity of your fear. Unfortunately, there are times in our lives when it is certainly appropriate to be afraid but it never serves you to be disempowered. You can escape from a dangerous situation while maintaining a semblance of control. The key is to keep a clear head. This may open up other avenues of dealing with the situation, which panic might cause you to miss.

Most of us take breathing for granted. We don't give it a thought unless our air supply is somehow compromised. Yet the quality of our breathing has an important impact on our health. Efficient breathing better oxygenates our blood. This means that our brains and internal organs receive more oxygen and work more effectively. The way we breathe affects our emotions as well. When we want to calm ourselves, we breathe deeply, allowing the chest and abdomen to move with the diaphragm, which is the primary muscle for breathing. When you breathe in, the chest and abdomen move outward. When you breathe out, the chest and abdomen relax back into place.

When we are responding out of fear, whether it's fear for our physical safety or emotional turmoil, we start to breathe high up in the chest—short, shallow breathing. This type of breathing signals the body that it's time either to fight or to flee. The body starts pumping adrenaline, and our muscles contract to be ready for action. This response in turn makes us feel agitated and even more short of breath. These reactions all translate into feeling emotionally upset and afraid.

Here is a way to use breath to regulate an emotional reaction:

The moment you start to feel upset, stop and take a deep, full breath all the way from the chest into the abdomen. Slow, deep, full breathing signals the body that it can relax. Automatically, the interplay between your breath and your body allows you to calm down so that you can think more clearly.

To illustrate this concept, try a simple exercise:

Start to breathe shallowly up in the chest, taking short quick breaths. The only part of your body that moves with your breath should be the top of the chest. Keep breathing like this and be aware of how you start to feel emotionally. You will most likely begin to feel upset for no apparent reason *because this is what your body is telling you*. Now, start to slow your breath, breathing deeply all the way into the abdomen, so that both the chest and the stomach move with your breath. As you slow and deepen your breath, your mind and emotions will also relax. You will notice the anxiety leaving not only your body, but your mind as well.

The following exercise also illustrates the connection of breath, body, and mind:

Think of something that you *were* upset about but were able to resolve. Put yourself back in time and allow yourself to feel all the accompanying emotions of the situation *before* you solved the problem. Remember how you felt. Notice that as you relive the discomfort of this emotional incident, your breathing becomes shallower, moving higher up into your chest.

Now, remind yourself that the troublesome aspect of this circumstance has been remedied. As you feel relief, notice that your breathing has gone back to normal.

Go back to the first step in this exercise, and instead of using your thoughts to calm you, just alter your breathing. Start to take deep, full breaths and notice that your mind automatically responds. Your feeling of anxiety will diminish as well.

These are very simple techniques to see how we unconsciously listen to the signals of our bodies. In one exercise, we used the mind to decrease anxiety.

In the other exercises, we used the breath, not the intellect, to calm down. These are examples of how we can start with the body to still our minds and begin to regain our power.

Breathing is the *most* basic Power Practice. The moment you relinquish your energy, stop for a moment and regulate your breathing to clear your head and calm yourself. This sets the stage for any Power Practice. Always start by taking a deep breath.

Chapter 5

POWER IN PRESENT TIME

Every instant that we are not conscious in the present moment, whether we are worrying about the future or ruminating about the past, we are not fully living our lives. If we're worried that we won't be happy tomorrow, next month, or next year, or if we are angry that we weren't happy in the past, then we are never truly happy. When we are stuck in the past, concerned with people or incidents that we can't let go of, or when we are worried and anxious about the future, we are not fully in our power. We are not living our lives *now,* when it counts. We are sending our chi back into the past and forward into the future, rather than being in our power in the present moment. Therefore, our power is diluted over the years of our life, rather than concentrated here and now, when we need it. When we are present in the moment, we are also living in the energy of love, because we aren't angry about the past and worried about what's to come.

It is always possible, of course, that there is something really frightening happening in the present moment, and it may be appropriate to be afraid or angry. Being in your power means that you can move through your fear-based emotions and not get stuck in them. It is also possible that your fear is not actually about what is happening now but results from your anticipation of some future event or inability to let go of a past trauma. If this is the case, you are not in your power. Practicing these exercises will give you the skills to manage your chi to your best advantage, empowering you to deal most effectively with any situation.

The following exercise helps you call back your chi from the past or future and plug it into the present moment. When you first try this, take your time. As you practice it, you will be able to perform this exercise in a matter of seconds.

You don't have to memorize the exact words of any of these practices to get their full benefit. Power in Present Time is a useful tool to begin any meditation set forth in this book.

Power in Present Time

1. Lie down in a comfortable position, making sure that your spine is straight. Close your eyes. Take a deep breath.

2. Imagine that your energy is an electrical cord that can plug into different people and situations. Imagine, too, that every breath you take pulls in radiant, healing light. With every breath, that light penetrates deeper and deeper into every single cell of your body. As you relax more and more,

let go until there is no tension anywhere in your body. Soon you are completely relaxed.

3. Take this moment to call your chi, your thoughts, your emotions back
from all that occurred in your past.

4. Unplug your energy, your spirit, your thoughts from your past with
gratitude for its gifts and lessons.

5. Acknowledge that the past is what carried you to this point in your life.
Call your chi into this moment, affirming that the past is over.

6. Unplug your energy from your worries for the future.

Remember that you are exactly where you're meant to be.

7. Call your life force energy back from the future, into this moment.

8. Feel the power of being fully present, here and now.

9. Memorize this feeling of being present and in your power. How does it
feel? How does your body feel? What is the rhythm of your breath? Feel
the vibration of your total body chi. When you are ready, open your eyes,
maintaining this feeling of conscious awareness.

You can use the following as a short practice the instant you realize that
you are not present in the moment:

Take a deep breath and imagine that you are pulling all your energy plugs
from the past and the future. Move your mental focus into the present by feeling your chi return to you. Feel the chi throughout your whole body.

An essential aspect of this exercise is expressed by the phrase "You are exactly
where you're meant to be." According to the belief system that inspires Chi

Fitness, all human beings incarnate on Earth to learn and experience specific lessons so that our souls can evolve. Wherever you are in your life right now is perfect for you to learn what you need to learn.

Another aspect of Power in Present Time is trusting that tomorrow will take care of itself. This can be hard to embrace when you have children to organize and bills to pay. It doesn't mean you should ignore your obligations or avoid making preparations for the future. It simply means to keep your power in present time as much as possible. This will help you manage your energy and accomplish what you need to do on a daily basis.

Before you begin a meditation, you want to have as much chi in the present moment as possible. Only then is it available for you to manage with your thoughts and intentions. This practice is important and serves as the beginning of every other meditation in this book. Remember that you can pull your power into present time in a single moment once you become familiar with this technique.

You will find that some meditations begin with an abbreviated form of this short practice: "Call your energy, your spirit, your thoughts back from everything that is not here and now." Note that for every power practice, all the steps will be listed so you never have to page back to previous chapters.

Addendum to Power in Present Time
Experiencing Power Loss

1. Once you have experienced your power in present time, memorize that feeling. Imprint the sensation in your body and mind.

2. Picture in your mind's eye a person who infuriates you. Allow yourself to experience all the emotions that accompany your perception of this person. Don't stop your feelings; let them flow.

3. Draw your attention to how your body feels when you are giving away your chi in this manner. You may feel off-balance, or you may feel discomfort in a particular area of your body.

4. Contrast this feeling with the one you had when you were in your power. Memorize what relinquishing your chi feels like so that when this happens, you will immediately recognize it.

If you are having trouble picturing a person who angers you, there are many techniques to trigger an emotional memory. You do it every day without thinking about it, but trying to have the experience when you want may prove difficult. You can use any of your senses to retrieve a memory. Some people find it easiest to see an image in their mind's eye, but you may need to rely on your other senses, recalling a smell, taste, feel, or sound to evoke an emotional memory. If this process continues to be frustrating, you can find an actual picture of the person you're thinking of and use that for this exercise. Explore what works best for you.

You may think that you are fully present without really being so. Most of us are not used to disciplining our energy. You can be worrying about what you have to do next or comparing today to yesterday without even being conscious of it. Practicing Power in Present Time gives you the experience of truly being in your power, because you are consciously letting go of both the past and the future. In this practice you are *physically* experiencing what it is like to be in charge of your energy by pulling it into the present. This practice is also important because it's impossible to have the physical realization of relinquishing your power unless you know what being in your power feels like.

Power in Present Time and Experiencing Power Loss are exercises that allow you to internalize what being empowered and disempowered feel like. Commit to memory the physical experience of each so that when you give your chi away, you will immediately perceive it and take steps to recover your energy.

Chapter 6

RECLAIMING YOUR CHI

You will probably use this technique more often than any other. Once you become familiar with what it feels like to be in your power, you will realize when you have given it away. That is when you will use the Power Practice, Reclaiming Your Chi. This practice is the actual pulling back of your chi. It builds on the practice, Power in Present Time. When you are relinquishing your chi, you are, in effect, sending your chi outside yourself. You might be attaching your energy to other people's behavior in a way that undermines your self-confidence, or you could be trying to control something over which you have no control. This is fear-based behavior that disempowers you.

Power in Present Time is a general Power Practice that gathers your energy into the moment. Reclaiming Your Chi is more specific to particular instances of giving away your power. You will feel as if you have cast out a fishing line and now are reeling it back in, pulling back a piece of yourself into your energy system. The act of taking back your chi leaves you feeling energized, grounded, and calm.

If you are wondering how you can be energized and calm at the same time, contrast this state of being to nervous energy, which is more of a hindrance than a help to you. Usually if you are filled with nervous energy, it is due to some underlying anxiety. Energized calm is one aspect of feeling empowered. It fills you with exhilaration, while you remain serene and content, without feeling as though you are going to jump out of your skin.

The following exercise teaches you how to reclaim your chi in any situation.

Reclaiming Your Chi

1. Lie down in a comfortable position, making sure that your spine is straight. Take a deep breath. Close your eyes. Call your energy, your spirit, your thoughts back from everything that is not here and now.

2. Be aware of your deep, full breathing. Be aware of your body. Be aware of the chi running through your body. Finally, be aware of the feeling of being fully in your power in this moment.

3. Picture in your mind's eye a person to whom you have given your power. Feel and identify the accompanying emotions. Whether it is anger you're feeling or shame or jealousy, remember that fear is the root emotion. Notice how you feel in your body as you give away your energy to these feelings.

4. Understand that on the energetic level you are sending out lines of energy, just like a fishing line that hooks into the object of your negative emotions. You are disempowering yourself.

5. Visualize these energy lines going from your body and hooking into the person you are imagining. See your energy as brilliant white light within you and surrounding you.

6. Picture yourself unhooking your energy out of that individual and back to you, just as easily as you would reel in a fishing line.

7. Keep in mind that this is within your power. Energy follows thought and intention, and you are in control of it. Feel now that you are once again fully present and in your power. Feel the surge of energy that occurs in your entire body when you take your power back.

If you can't visualize the lines of chi leaving your body, allow the visualization of energy cords leaving your body to come to you naturally. Don't try to control what that visualization looks like. You already *unconsciously* know where your energy is. Trust whatever picture comes into your mind and go on with the exercise.

It is important to remember that when we reclaim our chi from someone, we are not abandoning him or sapping his energy. We are allowing him to be in his own power, just as we are empowering ourselves.

You may be pulling your chi back from someone who is accustomed to controlling you. In that case, as he feels you disengaging, he may double his effort at domination. In a situation like this, continue to stay in your power. As long as you don't participate in this other person's fear-based behavior, you won't relinquish your chi. Having compassion for his frustration will empower you further, and ideally it will inspire him as well.

You may feel concerned that taking back your energy from an individual might deplete his power. In reality, you are doing him a service because you are taking back your chi, empowering yourself, and allowing him to be in his own power. It is important to remember that you can never take another person's chi. You are the only one who controls your energy. You may give your power away to somebody by allowing her to control you, but that does not empower her. Even if this person has you completely under her thumb, she is disempowered, because by controlling you, she is invested in your behavior. Therefore, this person has relinquished her chi just as much as you have. Whenever you try to control something that you ultimately have no control over—such as another person's behavior—you are giving away your power.

Often another concern that someone will voice is that if he takes his power back from someone he loves he may be abandoning her. For example, a friend may be going through a divorce. You are helping her as much as you can, but you feel that the extent of your involvement is becoming unhealthy for both of you. She is becoming so overly demanding and jealous of your time that your life is being seriously affected by her extreme neediness. You feel conflicted because you want to put up a boundary, but you keep getting sucked into her hysterical behavior. When you reclaim your chi from your friend, you are able to set healthy limits in the time you spend with her, but you still question whether you have abandoned her. The answer is that you are staying in your power and allowing her to be in hers. In fact, when you reclaim your chi, the resulting energetic shift can also cause a positive shift in her behavior, inspiring her to reclaim her chi as well. Your empowerment ultimately serves everyone around you.

Short Practice

If you feel that you're losing energy, simply imagine that you are pulling all your energy back into your body. Picture your energy as brilliant white light within and around you. Visualize where you have attached your chi. Take a deep breath and pull your energy back to you. You will immediately feel more grounded, centered, and powerful.

Chapter 7

LETTING GO OF FEAR

Letting Go of Fear is a Basic Power Practice that helps you dissolve anxiety. Any time you are feeling an emotion that is not love, you are actually experiencing fear. Remember that if you're angry, you're really afraid; if you're judging someone, you are really afraid; if you're jealous, that's fear, too. Fear leaves you powerless.

Many people believe that the soul creates circumstances in your life that bring your fears to the surface. When you are afraid of something or someone, the fear is usually due to emotional wounding in the past. In order to heal these fears, you must first experience, then acknowledge them. Instead of fighting your fears and pushing them down into your subconscious, you can learn to embrace and heal them.

The body stores all of your experiences, thoughts, and feelings. Fear will manifest as a block in the area of the body governed by a specific chakra. This information will be covered in greater detail in Part III. For now, don't worry about *why* a fear manifests in a certain area of your body. Just identify where it is. Remember not to judge yourself as you explore your fears. Rely on your intuition to guide you through the exercises.

When a fear-based emotion overcomes you, this practice will help you learn to dissolve it and replace it with love.

Letting Go of Fear

1. Lie down in a comfortable position with your spine straight and relaxed. Take a deep breath. Close your eyes.

2. Unplug from everything that is not here and now. Call your energy, your spirit, your thoughts back from the past with gratitude for its gifts and lessons.

3. Call your energy, your spirit, your thoughts back from your worries about the future, remembering that you are exactly where you're meant to be.

4. Take a few moments to get in touch with your body, your chi, your breath. Recognize the feeling of being fully in your power, in this moment.

5. Think of what you are afraid of in your life right now and allow yourself to feel all the upset that goes with it.

6. Identify the place in your body where the fear is most intense. It could be in your throat, your stomach, your forehead, your lower back, or any combination of these. There is no *wrong* answer. Trust your perception of where your fear lies.

7. Put your awareness in that spot and give the fear shape and color in your mind's eye.

8. Realize that this fear is a part of you. Think of it in a new way: Instead of something that has to be battled against, think of it as a child you have created to teach you an important lesson. This child is afraid and needs love and nurturing.

9. Comfort this fear just as you would your own child. Send gratitude for the lessons it carries. Send light and love to that place in your body. As you nurture it, watch as the color of fear fades and is replaced by the brilliant white light of love.

10. Take a moment to acknowledge the perfect, beautiful light that is all of you. Take a deep breath and open your eyes, knowing that at any time you can replace your fear, your darkness, with love and light.

When you practice Letting Go of Fear, you will learn to identify what fear feels like in your body. You will know that you have released your fear when you are again confronted with the same issue and it evokes no physical or emotional charge. There will be no sense of energy loss.

Keep in mind that this is a process. Fear often has many layers and dissipating it can take time, but each time your reaction will be more empowered than before. Nurture yourself in this journey. It is important to realize that many of our fears are deep-seated, and releasing them is a process requiring practice.

One of the keys to letting go of fear is the simple act of acknowledging it and then exploring its roots. Our instinct is usually to hide from our fears or to wage war against them. Battling against an emotion is, in itself, fear-based behavior. Fighting an emotion causes you to feel even more fearful. Acknowledging your fear automatically starts to empower you. It's like the old joke "Don't think about pink elephants." Once you hear that phrase, *all* you can do is visualize pink elephants. The harder you try *not* to think of them, the stronger the images become in your mind. On the other hand, if you just say to yourself, "All I can think about are pink elephants," and allow yourself to visualize them, soon you will be able to forget the whole silly thing. The same scenario occurs when we try to hide from our panic. It's all we can think about—and the anxiety grows. When you admit your fear, then go a step further and *embrace* it, this act of nurturing empowers you to let it go.

Consider this as another example of why battling your fear doesn't work. If you're jealous of another person, you may have a fear of inadequacy. Obsessing over your feelings only causes you to become more jealous and afraid. But if you verbalize, "I'm really feeling jealous of this person because deep down I feel totally inadequate," you will have already started to take the power out of your fear. The act of admitting your fear moves it into the open, so you can use the power practices for self-healing. The act of acknowledging and expressing your feelings allows you to nurture yourself and reclaim the chi you had given away.

A Personal Note

All my life I have struggled with abandonment issues that are linked to feelings of inadequacy. In the past, my relationships with men always reflected this general theme. I believed that I wanted true intimacy in a relationship, but this always seemed to elude me. What I now realize is that my relationships were not intimate because I was not capable of having intimacy. I would always think that I just "chose the wrong man," when really the lack of closeness in each relationship occurred because I didn't have a clue as to what real intimacy was between a man and a woman—and I attracted partners who reflected this back to me. I enjoyed intimate relationships with women, but never with men.

I was thirty-five, with two beautiful children and in my second marriage, before I started on a spiritual quest. I went into therapy and did a lot of work on myself. My husband and I grew apart. We divorced amicably and established a solid, cooperative relationship as joint parents. Shortly thereafter, I fell madly in love with another man. In this relationship, I thought I had found the closeness I craved. We were together for three years, but our relationship ended abruptly when I was dumped unceremoniously for another woman. I was crushed. All my abandonment issues and feelings of insignificance and inadequacy came screaming to the surface. I know now that this experience occurred to spur my growth. The intensity of the breakup offered me a spiritual opportunity. Without it, I never would have discovered the roots of these issues and started a healing process.

About a year after this traumatic episode, I met Drew. Here was a man who was eager and able to enter an intimate relationship—yet as much as I liked him, he frightened me. I realized that my feelings came from my own fear of intimacy, but I wondered what was wrong with *him* because he so obviously admired me. My self-esteem was clearly not in a healthy state. By admitting to myself how scared I was, I could face my fears and start to do the work I needed to reclaim my chi. Drew moved in with me and my two children, and we were very happy. I felt that he was my best friend and our relationship was joyful and fulfilling. Drew wanted to get married. I was leery, but willing. Around the time that we were going to send out wedding invitations, I started getting cold feet. We were so happy the way we were. What if marriage changed everything? I had been married *twice* already. Was I crazy to do it again? I was in a state of panic. I knew I had to say something to Drew, but I was afraid he would get angry and leave me. These primal fears of abandonment were totally unfounded in the context of our relationship, but my experience with significant others (including my parents) had rarely given me space to feel entitled to voice negative feelings. I pushed these emotions down, making my anxiety even more intense, visualizing the worst possible scenes in my mind until I thought I'd explode. One night, my fear manifested itself as a painful constriction in my throat and heart area, making it impossible for me to conceal my feelings any longer. I screwed up my nerve and confessed my terror to Drew. As soon as I openly acknowledged my fears, I could feel the chi I had been blocking rush through me, carrying with it immense relief. I found that the very moment I acknowledged and embraced my fear, I could let go of it. I told Drew the reasons I was afraid to get married again. As much as I loved him, I wasn't sure I could go through with the wedding. I asked him whether he would continue to live with me if we weren't married. His answer melted the ice around my heart. He lovingly let me know that he was disappointed and upset but would never leave me. He didn't try to manipulate or pressure me. Drew's response confirmed that entering into a partnership with him was a wonderfully right decision. In fact, we got married several months later. Happily, I don't even feel "married." I feel as if I'm living with my passionate, loving best friend.

Chapter 8

SPIRITUAL PERSPECTIVE

The basic belief behind the practice of Spiritual Perspective is that every circumstance in your life serves a higher purpose. Your soul creates experiences in order for your spirit to grow and learn.

Spiritual Perspective allows you to unplug your energy from people or situations and see your life from a higher place. This practice helps you see the larger picture, the *why* of what is happening in your life, without the confusion of fear-based emotional reactions.

Unplugging or reclaiming your chi will restore your power in any situation. Ultimately, you will use whatever Power Practices work best for you and come most naturally to you. Using Spiritual Perspective literally enables you to see the larger picture, helping you to figure out the *why* and *how* of any experience.

Picture yourself getting onto a Ferris wheel. Before it starts to move, you have the same perspective as everyone else on the ground. Once your chair lifts up, the higher you get the farther you can see. Things that would have blocked your perception suddenly shrink into insignificance, allowing you to perceive events that would otherwise have been beyond your frame of reference. Using Spiritual Perspective, you can see everything leading up to a particular event and all the circumstances surrounding it. You can pull your energy back from fear-based emotions evoked by any situation and empower yourself further by expanding your field of vision.

When you energetically remove yourself from an event in your life by rising above it, you have automatically unplugged from your fear. The absence of fear confirms that you are not fabricating this perspective. Perceiving with the eyes of your spirit clarifies the lessons you are meant to learn from any circumstance. *After all, you are not a physical being having a spiritual experience: you are a spiritual being having a physical experience.* Any time you are experiencing fear in any of its forms, you are not being your true self.

Your spirit is your true self, not your personality. When you are acting in alignment with your soul, you do not experience fear because your behavior is based in love. When you are afraid, you are disconnected from your spirit. Therefore, you are not being your true self. When you experience and embody love, you are allowing your spirit to lead you through the physical world.

It can seem the height of arrogance to ask people to accept that there is a higher purpose for their suffering. There are horrific incidents happening everywhere that are beyond human endurance and comprehension. What purpose could possibly be served by these abominations? And yet, the key to finding peace in the face of tragedy is just such a Spiritual Perspective. The point of this Power Practice is to help you unplug your energy from a traumatic situation and begin to experience the serenity that can come from finding something positive in what seems to be only negative. This doesn't mean that you shouldn't fully experience your grief. In fact, you have to experience your grief to move through it. The trap, as in any fear-based emotion, is getting stuck in it. This practice can help you find solace when it seems unattainable.

If an event is so awful that you find it impossible to look at—from any perspective—let your point of view continue to rise above the situation, getting as high or far away as you need to. Don't think about or judge the process. You may end up in outer space or on a South Sea island. Whatever comes up for you can lead to psychological, emotional, and spiritual insights. As with all of these power practices, the *physical* experience of managing your chi precedes any intellectual examination of what transpires.

Spiritual Perspective

1. Get into a comfortable sitting position. Straighten the spine by lifting up through the crown of the head and gently pushing downward through the tailbone. Take a deep breath. Close your eyes.

2. Call your energy, your spirit, your thoughts back from everything that is not here and now. Be aware of the feeling of being fully in your power in this moment.

3. In your mind's eye, picture a person or situation that is upsetting you. Allow yourself to feel whatever emotions come up. Reclaim your chi by pulling your energy back to you.

4. Enjoy the feeling of being in your power. Then, with your thoughts and intentions, raise your energy up over your head and look down with the eyes of your spirit as if your physical body were elevated over the scene. From this point of view, energetically, you can see the situation from a higher viewpoint, a spiritual perspective.

5. Look at the scene from above and examine the events leading up to this point in time. You have an expanded view and can see the larger picture.

6. Ask yourself, "What is the lesson here? What is the gift?" See whether, from this higher perspective, you can discern the purpose of this scenario.

7. If you can't find a lesson, see whether you can trust that there *is* a purpose, even if it's not clear to you now. By disengaging your energy from the situation and projecting your chi upward, you have unplugged from the emotion the circumstances provoked.

8. Pull your chi back down to your body. Think about what you have learned by changing your perspective.

It may be that doing this practice allows you to perceive an aspect of the scenario that you had not been aware of before. This may arouse a fear-based reaction. If this is the case, you can use the practice, Reclaiming Your Chi or Letting Go of Fear. You can also ask yourself the Four Questions for Healing to identify the roots of your disturbance and which chakra is relinquishing chi. (This topic will be explored in the next chapter.) Performing these practices will help you approach this situation from a point of power, without fear.

Short Practice

Once you have become familiar with Spiritual Perspective, you can do it in a moment. When you want to know *why* you are facing a particular circumstance, take a deep breath and mentally rise above the scene to look down on it. Ask yourself, "What is the lesson here? What is really going on?" See whether an answer comes to you. Even if you can't see the meaning in it, you will have reminded yourself that every situation serves a purpose in your life.

Allison's Experience

Allison learned the Power Practices just before there was a family gathering at her home. Ever since Allison and her older sister, Joy, were children, Allison would give away her power to Joy, who is very overbearing. Joy is still very critical of Allison, and Joy's remarks would cause her to feel inferior. Using these Power Practices has caused two things to happen in the sisters' relationship. Allison recognized that Joy's behavior toward her is based in jealousy—which Allison now knows is fear. Once Allison realized this, she could feel compassion for Joy, instead of anger. This has changed the energy of their relationship in a positive way. Joy doesn't seem to be so critical anymore. There *are* times when Joy can "get to" Allison, and Allison gives her power away to Joy, but now Allison has the tools to reclaim her chi. After practicing these techniques only a few times, taking back her energy became second nature to Allison. Pulling back her power now seems to happen the instant she thinks about it.

Jenny's Experience

Jenny and her boss don't get along at all. Jenny is the only woman in the upper management of her company, and her position sets off a lot of hidden and not-so-hidden resentment. She went to a business meeting in California, expecting to have a very difficult time, as usual—but found that she could use these Power Practices to keep her energy with her the entire time, without being drawn into any political infighting. When she started to feel upset and angry, she realized immediately when she was giving her power away. She visualized the energy cords attaching outside herself and just "pulled the plug," disengaging from her fear. Jenny felt calm and relaxed and could distance herself from the situation—participating fully in her work without being distracted by the pettiness of office politics.

Chapter 9

FOUR QUESTIONS FOR HEALING AND SELF-TALK

As you begin the journey of self-awareness through managing your chi, several things will become clearer to you. You will begin to realize which people and situations are most likely to provoke you to give away your power. You will see patterns in your life that you were not aware of before. You might notice repeating scenarios that seem old and familiar, even though the players may change. You may want to moderate your emotional reaction to a certain person or alter the outcome of a recurring conflict.

You may find yourself asking, "Why is this happening again?" or "Why does this person make me crazy?" When you use the Four Questions for Healing, you will be able to recognize what in your past is similar to a present situation in which you lose your power.

For example, there may be an individual in your life who riles you, even though you can't explain why this person bugs you so much. In all probability, you had a troubled relationship with someone in your past whose energy was similar to this individual's, and you are unconsciously making a connection between that person in the past and this person now.

The same kind of connection can lead to attraction instead of repulsion. It is common for people who grow up around addicts to marry or have serious relationships with substance abusers later in life. When a pattern like this occurs, you need to get to the root of why you are attracted to people who replay the same negative circumstances you've endured before. These individuals appear in your life to give you the opportunity to heal the fear-based emotions that you experienced in your past. If you don't heal the wound with *this* person, your spirit will lead you to *another* until you succeed in taking back your power.

Remember that there is a purpose for everything that happens in your life. People and situations stir up charged emotions rooted in the past so that you can work on healing them now.

Your soul manifests situations that draw your wounds to the surface in order to be healed. For example, if you are sensitive to judgment, you will continue to attract criticism (or what *feels* like criticism) until you take steps to resolve the issues underlying your sensitivity.

If you don't feel comfortable delving into your past, you can use the Power Practices to keep pulling your energy back from a particular individual or circumstance. Over time, it will become second nature to you and you will be able to unplug instantly.

However, all experiences that give you an emotional charge can be used to heal your childhood wounds, and repeatedly unplugging your chi from a particular person or event is not going to help you heal. The universe will continue to present you with more opportunities to address the very wound you don't want to examine. You might as well look into your past now.

If you are dealing with a very deep wound, these questions may uncover feelings that you have trouble dealing with on your own. You may then want to seek out a therapist who can support and facilitate your journey within. Professionals can guide you through your past in a way that will nurture you and assuage your fear. In the meantime, you can use the Power Practices and self-talk to unplug from your anxiety.

All of the Basic Power Practices, the Four Questions for Healing, and self-talk will come into play to start you on your healing path. Use the Four Questions when you relinquish your power repeatedly in similar circumstances. If you find yourself having to unplug from a particular individual all the time, there is something in your relationship with this person that you need to explore. Otherwise, you will find yourself constantly pulling your chi back from her without really healing the underlying wound that causes you to react the way you do. The same thing can happen with recurring situations. Say you are frequently enraged by other drivers' tailgating you. The next time this happens, you have several choices when you get angry. You can give your power away by changing your speed in reaction to the other driver—accelerating to stay ahead or slowing down to obstruct him. If this is a frequent scenario in your life, you would benefit from asking yourself the Four Questions. On the other hand, if you can pull over and choose to let the other driver pass without "rising to the bait," you have taken your power back by not getting stuck in your anger. Metaphorically speaking, by pulling your car over you have literally pulled your anger out of the situation; by letting the driver pass, you are letting your anger pass by. When you can handle a problem this way, you don't need to analyze it any further with the Four Questions. Whenever you overreact and give away your power, ask yourself the following questions:

Four Questions for Healing

1. The moment I relinquished my chi, how old did I feel?
2. What happened when I was that age?
3. How is that past situation similar to the current one?
4. When I have an emotional reaction about this situation, where do I feel it in my body?

Once you have answered these questions, you can use the Basic Power Practices and self-talk to begin your healing work.

When you use these Four Questions you will discover the origin of your behavior, which is usually rooted in childhood. Your task is to heal yourself and take your power back, using the Basic Power Practices and self-talk. Note that there is a distinction between self-talk and the inner dialogue that we carry on with ourselves all day long. Talking to yourself is often an unconscious habit. It can be a very destructive one, too. Most of us wouldn't abuse our worst enemies with the cruel things we routinely say to ourselves. Self-talk as described in this book is consciously treating yourself in a loving, nurturing, and respectful way. It helps you take care of yourself on a deep level.

One of the most important benefits of self-talk is that it helps you tell yourself what you needed to hear (but didn't) in childhood. Maybe your four-year-old self needs to know that the illness in your family was not her responsibility. Or the twelve-year-old needs to hear how creative he is. Even as an adult, you need to give yourself words of encouragement and learn to be a parent and best friend to yourself.

Think about how you talk to yourself. It is important to learn to treat yourself as you would a beloved child or dear friend. Engaging in this behavior will empower you.

There are many reasons we give up our power. They usually have to do with the behavior patterns we learned as children that helped us to survive in our family of origin. These patterns don't necessarily continue to serve us as adults, and we must find a way to heal the wounds that cause the type of behavior we want to stop.

For example, say you're at a dinner party and you have expressed an opinion. Your host rudely laughs it off, telling you that your remark is ridiculous. You immediately feel crushed; in fact, you feel as though you've been punched in the solar plexus. You realize that you have given your chi away, and you use a short practice in the moment to reclaim your power—but you still have more work to do.

When circumstances appear in your life that push your buttons, there is a reason. The purpose is to draw your wounds to the surface to be acknowledged and then healed. *When you heal yourself, you are reclaiming your chi from old scenarios that have continued to affect how you choose to live your life.* When you heal those wounds, you are revitalizing important parts of your energy system so that it can operate at full power.

Let's return to the dinner party where the host scoffs at your opinion. You feel ridiculed and very upset. You ask yourself, "Why do I react so violently when this kind of a situation occurs?" (Since you are sensitive to criticism, you can bet you get a lot of it.) This is where the Power Practices come in. You can use a short practice to take your power back right away. Later, you can revisit the scene in your head and ask yourself the Four Questions for Healing and use self-talk.

Before asking yourself the first question, take a deep, full, long breath. Then draw your chi into the moment by using Power in Present Time. Call your energy, your spirit, your thoughts back from everything that is not here and now. Feel the power of being fully present in this moment.

Now ask yourself the first question: "The moment I relinquished my chi, how old did I feel?" Trust that the first answer that pops into your head is the right one.

Explore that by asking yourself, "What happened when I was that age?" Using Spiritual Perspective, project your energy upward and look down on your life. See yourself at that age and look at the conditions that surrounded you. Put yourself in that child's body, into the same environment, and see what happened. What was going on in your home life at that point? In this example, you might remember that your parents were having a rough spot in their marriage when you were six years old.

The third question is, "How is that past situation similar to the current one?" Still using Spiritual Perspective to rise above your body, see your past and present life from a higher point of view. How does the past situation compare to the present one (your distress at the dinner party)?

You may recall that the dinner table was a place where your parents openly sparred. Any time you tried to talk at the table, tensions ran so high that your parents were quick to criticize and contradict just about everything you said, or so it appeared to you. This contributed to your feelings of inadequacy. Children, of course, internalize so much, so intensely, and often feel responsible for what is going on around them. They can internalize guilt for their parents' divorce or for any abuse they themselves have suffered. Every stage in our lives is crucial to the soul's development, but childhood is especially critical because that is when we develop our personalities and ways of coping with life.

The comments of the dinner party host are especially provocative because they evoke the same feelings you had as a child. In this example, the scene is a direct parallel of the past. However, a situation doesn't have to be similar; it just has to evoke the same *feelings*. If you think there is a connection between what is happening now and a specific incident in your past, *there is*, even if it isn't obvious to your conscious mind. Keep exploring the connection and trust your instincts.

The fourth question is, "When I have an emotional reaction about this situation, where do I feel it in my body?" When you initially ask yourself this question, you can lie on the floor in a relaxed position with your spine straight. Draw your chi into present time by calling your energy, your spirit, your thoughts into this moment. Be aware of your total body chi and relax fully into the floor. Now allow yourself to feel the emotions of your past and present in relation to the situation you are now exploring. Where do you feel these emotions most intensely? Visualize that part of your body.

Here you have a choice about which practice to use: Letting Go of Fear or Reclaiming Your Chi, or both, in addition to self-talk. Always start by taking a deep, full, long breath. You can use the Letting Go of Fear practice by giving a color to the place in your body where you feel the emotions in question. Recognize that this is where your fear has manifested itself. Give the fear shape and color in your mind's eye.

Realize that this fear is a part of you. Feel gratitude for the lessons it carries. Send light and love to that place in your body. As you nurture yourself, watch as the color of fear fades and is replaced by the brilliant white light of love.

You can also use the practice Reclaiming Your Chi, by itself or in addition to Letting Go of Fear. Visualize the energy cords leaving your body wherever you feel an emotional charge. These cords connect to the past and present situations. Send love and light to the past and present, including the people involved. Now simply "pull the plug." Call your energy away from those people and circumstances, pulling your chi back to you.

By using self-talk you can place yourself in the position of a protector and nurturer of this child who was (and is) you. Mentally give him love and light, just as you would your own child who has been hurt. Say all the things to yourself as a child that you would say to a child of your own. Say to yourself *now* what you needed to hear *then*. This paves the way for healing old wounds. Self-talk and self-parenting can pull your energy from the past into present time, helping you feel safe enough to grow with confidence, faith, and love.

Just as chi can get stuck in your body, energy can get stuck in patterns of behavior that therapists call *core scenes*. For readers who don't know, a core scene is a series of events that you and a significant other act out repeatedly. For example, your husband may continually complain that you are never home from work in time for dinner. You agree to try to adjust your schedule so that you can have dinner together. The next night, you are home in time, but your husband stays out late, missing the meal you have prepared. The resulting argument doesn't resolve anything. You retaliate by not getting home by dinnertime for a week. Your husband complains again and negative feelings build up to the boiling point, causing serious damage to your relationship.

To change this core scene, you must both recognize when it occurs and choose to react differently the next time it does. Once you have taken this step, you can independently ask yourselves the Four Questions to get at the root of your behavior. You can then share your insights and work together to unplug from the past events that drive the fear-based behavior you want to stop.

Joanne's Experience

Joanne's mother was extremely controlling and self-centered. In fact, she probably had a Narcissistic personality disorder. As a child, Joanne was emotionally terrorized. She always felt she was "not good enough" if she did something that didn't meet with her mother's approval. Her mother would make her feel like such a bad child that it destroyed Joanne's self-esteem. Even as an adult, she had a self-image so shattered that she thought her dreams and desires must be wrong. The only way she could do what she wanted was never to share her true motives. When Joanne was a child, this was what worked in Joanne's family, what allowed her to survive, what saved her from relentless humiliation. As Joanne became an adult, it was a source of misery. She didn't know how to show anyone who she really was. Joanne could never genuinely, directly ask for what she wanted and needed. It had been drilled into her head that who she was wasn't good enough. This wound was so deep and Joanne was so unaware of its consequences that she never had a truly intimate relationship with anyone. She didn't know how to be herself.

In Joanne's case, when she enters into a relationship that has the potential for intimacy, she must recognize that the familiar feeling of fear is the signal that she is giving her power away. Once she is aware of this, she can ask herself the Four Questions. They will reveal to her the source of her anxiety, rooted in the past. Clearly, Joanne's wounding occurred early in her childhood. With the information she elicits from the Four Questions, she can use the Power Practices and take care of herself the way she should have been as a child. She can talk to herself as that four-year-old. If she doesn't know what to say to herself, she can imagine what she would say to a beloved child or a dear friend in such a situation. In this way, Joanne can begin to heal herself and establish relationships with a sense of trust and self-confidence.

PART III

Chakra Power Practices

The Basic Power Practices help you reclaim your energy once you have given away your power. As you become proficient at feeling your chi, you will be able to pinpoint where on your body you are losing energy. Once you understand where the energy loss is occurring, you can connect that place on your body with its corresponding energy center (*chakra*). Each chakra relates to a specific area of your life. By making the connection between a particular chakra and where you feel the energy leaving your body, you can explore why you are giving away your chi in that aspect of your life. The Chakra Power Practices build on the Basic Power Practices by enabling you to work with a specific chakra and a clearly defined issue in your life. For example, if you are using the Basic Power Practice Letting Go of Fear and you identify your fear as residing in the area of your solar plexus, you can use the technique for releasing your fear. Then, when you start working with your chakra system, you will recognize that since your fear is in the area of your solar plexus, which is the location of your third chakra, it means that you are dealing with an issue of self-esteem and the fear you are experiencing is affecting your self-image. You can start the healing process by using the Chakra Power Practices to unblock and manage your energy. Then you can utilize the Four Questions and self-talk for further exploration and growth.

Step 1 and Step 2 of the Chakra Power Practices are the same as the Basic Power Practices: being aware of your chi and perceiving that you have relinquished it.

Step 3 starts by associating that restriction or power loss with a particular energy center in your body. When you can sense where on your body you are losing energy, you can use the Basic Power Practice, Reclaiming Your Chi. To do this, imagine a brilliant cord of light radiating out from the place on your body that is relinquishing energy. This cord connects to something or someone outside yourself. Take a deep breath and pull the cord, just like an electrical wire, out of those people or situations that you are relinquishing your power to and reclaim your chi. Feel the energy surge that occurs when you call your chi back to you. If you want to do further work on unblocking and reclaiming your chi, you can use the Letting Go of Fear or Spiritual Perspective practices, depending on how you want to approach this exploration.

Step 3 also involves connecting the chakra where you are losing power with an aspect of your life. For instance, if you feel a weakness in the chest area, you are probably reacting to an issue regarding love and compassion, since any part of this area corresponds to the Heart Chakra. Trust your instincts.

Step 4 is using the Chakra Power Practices to unblock and manage your energy. You can use a Short Practice while the incident is occurring, and later refer to the exercises and meditations for the appropriate chakra.

In Step 5 you can use the Four Questions for Healing and self-talk, which will give you even more insight on your journey to empowerment.

For each Chakra Power Practice there will be a movement metaphor to connect the physical movement of each exercise to an aspect of your emotional life, as well as an affirmation that you can repeat to yourself throughout the day to help you remain empowered.

Chapter 10

OVERVIEW OF THE CHAKRAS

Chakra is a Sanskrit word that means, "wheel." The chakras are circular, spinning energy centers about the size of an orange located in the core of the body, from the tailbone through the crown of the head. They correspond to certain glands and organs that lie in proximity to each chakra. Each chakra also corresponds to a specific aspect of your life.

As in a person's aura, the colors of the chakras correspond to the elementary colors of the visible spectrum. Each color has a specific wavelength of light or energy frequency. Red has the longest wavelength, then orange, yellow, green, blue, indigo, and violet, which has the shortest wavelength. This natural order of colors is reflected in the order of chakras throughout the body.

The first chakra is located at the perineum, between the pubic bone and the tailbone. Its color is *red*. This is the root chakra. It is concerned with your family of origin, your "tribe," your background.

The second chakra is located between the pubic bone and navel. Its color is *orange*. This chakra is concerned with your creativity, sexuality, and external power in the world.

The third chakra is located at the solar plexus. Its color is *yellow*. This represents your self-esteem, your internal or authentic power.

The fourth chakra is located in the center of the chest, the heart center. Its color is *green*. This energy center is concerned with your love and compassion for yourself as well as for others.

The fifth chakra is located at the base of the throat. Its color is *blue*. This chakra is correlated to your will and speaking your truth.

The sixth chakra is located in the center of the forehead between the eyes—the "third eye." Its color is *indigo*. This chakra represents the power of the mind and intuition.

The seventh chakra is located at the crown of the head. Its color is *purple*. This center represents your connection with the divine.

As discussed in Chapter 1, colors in an energy field close to the body reflect your physical health, and colors perceived farther away from the body have to do with emotional and spiritual states. Just as a person's aura has many layers and shifting colors, each chakra is multilayered as well, with subtle variation in color reflecting different attitudes and moods and the state of a person's health. The complexity of this system should not inhibit you from trusting your own perception. Let your intuition guide you in this exploration.

Remember that this is not really an exercise of the mind; it is actually a process of letting go of the intellect, allowing your intuitive self to take over. Divine guidance is always available to you. You may believe that the source of this love and support is God or Nature or your Higher Self; that it is communicated to you by angels or nonphysical Teachers and Guides or by your instinct or intuition. However you conceive of it, your connection to a higher power is intrinsic to your state of being.

General Chakra Meditation

As you do this meditation, notice the vibrancy of the colors in each chakra. If any seems dull to you, look at the area in your life corresponding to that energy center and reflect upon it. For instance, if the yellow of your third chakra appears washed out, this may signal that a situation in your life is adversely affecting your self-esteem. If you can't perceive color clearly in your mind's eye, try sensing the energy in each center and intuit whether it is vibrant or blocked. Make these determinations without any sense of right or wrong, but with gentle nonjudgmental awareness.

1. Lie down, making sure that your spine is straight. A hard surface is better than a bed or a couch. Close your eyes, taking deep, full breaths.

2. Imagine that you are breathing in brilliant, radiant, clear, healing light that is streaming through your body, dissolving your tension and everyday worries.

3. As you breathe in more and more light, feel yourself becoming clearer, lighter, more radiant as you relax deeper and deeper, fully supported by the floor. Soon there is no tension anywhere in your body and you are completely relaxed.

4. Draw your attention to the area between your pubic bone and your tailbone. Sense the energy there. See whether you can visualize the color red. Remember, don't judge—just be aware of your impressions. Send the brilliant light in your body spiraling clockwise around this chakra. As you do, sense the light's becoming a more brilliant and radiant red, the energy more *alive*.

5. Progress to your second chakra and repeat the meditation, this time using the color orange.

6. Move through the rest of your chakra system:
- The third chakra is yellow.
- The fourth is green.
- The fifth is blue.
- The sixth is indigo.
- The seventh is purple. (See illustration.)

7. When you have gone through all the chakras, stay in your meditative state and be aware of the balance of your energy system, remembering that you are exactly where you're meant to be.

8. Remind yourself that you are always loved, supported, and guided on your journey. Take in a deep breath, then exhale. Whenever you feel ready, open your eyes.

You can then use one or all of the following movements in the next chapter to awaken and unblock your energy centers. Choose what appeals to you most. As you are doing the exercise, breathe through the energy center, visualizing the color for that chakra.

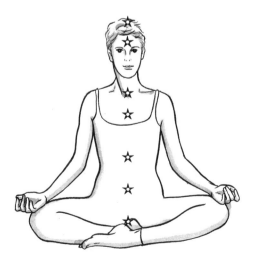

Chapter 11

CONSCIOUS MOVEMENT

onscious Movement is at the core of the Chakra Power Practices. Conscious Movement improves any kind of physical activity. It is movement that begins with *focus* and *intention* at a particular *point of power* within the body.

When moving consciously, visualize the point of power in your body and move from that place. For instance, if you're holding a free-weight and want to do a biceps curl, instead of just lifting the weight up to your shoulder by bending your elbow and raising your hand, consciously focus on the muscle, "seeing it" contract. Then, instead of just lowering the weight, visualize your biceps *expanding* as you lower the weight. Try it now: lift the palm of your hand to the front of your shoulder. This movement was just initiated from your hand. Now do the same movement, but this time lift your hand by contracting the biceps muscle. Feel the difference? Each of these is a conscious movement, with a different point of power. When the point of power is in the biceps, you're going to get a much better workout when you're lifting weights. Why? Because you're using intention and focus. You can *feel* that the muscle is working harder. Research has shown that if you use visualization with the intention of reshaping your physique, there can be significant changes in your body *even without exercise*. Obviously, if you exercise without using visualization, there will also be changes in your body, but if you use visualization along with working out, the results will be more powerful.

Remember: *energy follows intention* and your body is 99.9 percent energy. When you add conscious intention to the act of working out, you can get amazing results.

There are two basic forms of Conscious Movement: *core movement* and *external movement*.

Core movement has its point of power within the core of the body. External movement has its point of power outside the core of the body.

For example, say that an exercise calls for you to extend your arms away from your body, then slowly move your hands together in front of you. You could simply move your arms and hands. This would be an example of external movement, in which the origin of movement would be in your hands. Metaphorically speaking, sometimes it's necessary to "go gracefully" with the external events the universe presents to you.

An example of core movement would be to imagine that you have a hinge going down the middle of your body—a hinge that opens and closes both ways. By focusing on this hinge and contracting the muscles in the center of your chest, your hands would come together by using the muscles at the core of your body. In this example, the point of power is the center of your chest. The expansion and contraction of these muscles at your center allow energy to move more freely through your chakras. The flow of chi is unrestricted. Metaphorically, your life is inner-directed, guided by your feelings and intuition more than external influences.

Psychological and emotional tension can have a restricting effect on your energy system as well. Most people store tension in their bodies until it leads to illness or injury. These core movement exercises promote the free flow of chi through the parts of your body that correspond to each aspect of your life.

When you practice conscious movement, you begin to make connections in your mind about the mechanics of your body. You can feel what contraction in your body initiates what movement. Soon you are able to contract whatever muscle you want by merely putting your consciousness in that place. When this happens, you have much better familiarity with your body, and the quality of your physical activities improves. You acquire a finely attuned sensitivity to small changes in your physique, which helps you to head off illness. You will get signals from your body about your emotional well-being, too. The signs are most obvious when you experience a fear-based emotion: rapid, shallow breathing; increased heart rate; sweating; nausea. More extreme reactions range from rashes to panic attacks. On a subtler level, as you become more aware of how your body reflects your emotional state, you will be more sensitive to your energy system and better able to feel when and where you are giving away your chi. On the positive side, when you experience love-based emotions, your muscles are more relaxed, your heart rate slows down, and it is easier to take deep, full breaths. Your body feels vibrant and filled with energy.

When you use conscious movement, you'll be healthier because your chi will be circulating better. Before a disease manifests itself in your body, it starts at the energetic level when you continually give away your chi in a certain chakra. By using these practices, you will acquire a heightened perception of physical and energetic disorders, so you can stop an illness before it is expressed in the body in a serious way.

If you believe that disease begins energetically, then it follows that disease can be healed energetically as well. Throughout the ages, "energy medicine" has drawn upon the power of the body to heal itself when chi is set in bal-

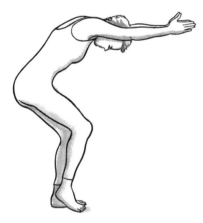

{ 1 }

ance. Western medicine has increasingly embraced "alternative" methods of healing to augment and, in some cases, supplant traditional treatment that may not be working effectively for a particular patient. What works best for you will be determined by your physical, emotional, psychological, and spiritual state of being.

Here are some core movement exercises for you to practice:

1. Start by facing front, arms stretched out to the sides at shoulder height. Your feet are in a wide stance, a little more than hip distance apart.

2. Visualize a hinge in the middle of your body. Contract from the center of the body, closing the hinge, moving the right side of the body to the left. To do this, you will keep the left side of your body stationary. When you close the hinge, turn the right side of your body to the left, moving the palms of your hands together while keeping your arms straight. At the same time, move your right leg to the left, knees bent slightly and touching. Let the head drop as you pull your arms and legs together.

{ 2 }

3. Open the hinge, using the core of the body to expand and open to center, facing forward.

4. Close your hinge so that you are facing to the right.

Expand the core of the body to center again. Visualize the hinge running through the middle of your body, closing and then opening, rather than simply letting the hands and arms move together and separate. Continue with these movements until you can really feel that the point of power for this exercise is in the center of your body.

You can also use core movement when you do sit-ups. In this example, you will work all of the abdominal muscles.

1. Lie down with your feet flat on the floor, knees up. Press your lower back into the floor and, before you do anything else, pull the abdominal muscles in, so that you have a "hollowed out" feeling in the stomach.

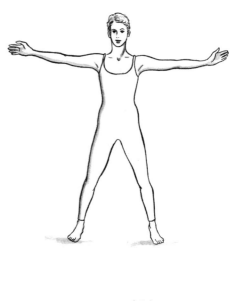

{ 3 }

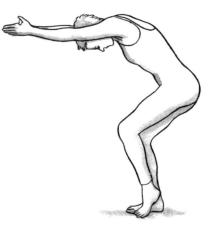

{ 4 }

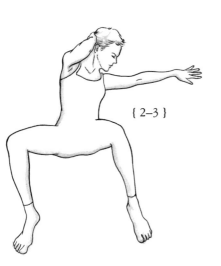

{ 2–3 }

2. Start with your left arm straight out to the side, left palm flat on the floor. Bend your right arm at the elbow with your right hand supporting your head.

3. Lift the right shoulder off the floor, aiming between the shoulder and the knee. This will work the muscles on the sides of the abdomen, in the waist. Holding this position, feel which muscles in your abdomen are contracting. Controlling the movement, slowly lower your shoulder back to the floor. Instead of initiating the movement from your shoulder, initiate the movement by contracting the muscles in the side of the abdomen. When you shorten this muscle group, the shoulder *must* lift up.

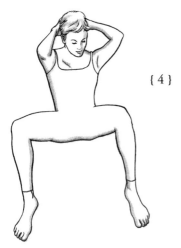

{ 4 }

4. Place both hands behind your head. (Always make sure you are not *pulling* the head, but supporting it.) Keeping your back pressed into the floor, lift your upper body toward the left knee. Feel exactly where your stomach is tightening, then use your intention to initiate the movement from the muscle in the left center of your stomach.

5. Lift your head and shoulders toward the space between your knees, engaging the muscles in the center of the stomach and allowing that contraction to lift your head and shoulders off the ground.

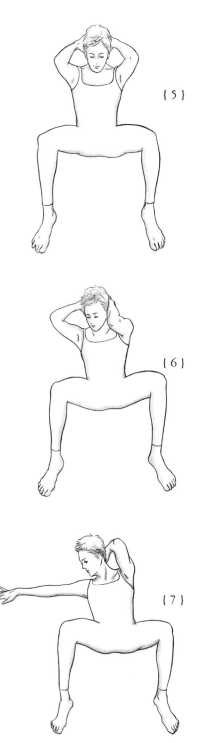

{ 5 }

6. Advance to the right center of the abdomen, lifting the body toward the right knee.

7. Finally, proceed by laying the right arm flat on the floor to stabilize the shoulder. Using the muscles at the right side of the abdomen, contract and lift your left shoulder all the way over between the right shoulder and knee.

For a great abdominal workout, do ten repetitions at each position. As you get stronger, you can increase the number of repetitions.

{ 6 }

Now, stay on your back with the lower back pressed into the floor. Without moving the upper body, see whether you can progress through each of these muscle groups by contracting them. First, take in a deep breath and place your awareness in the left side of the abdomen. Exhale as you squeeze the muscles there just as if you were lifting the shoulder. Then move to left center, center, right center, and right side. This exercise illustrates that with practice you can have control over every muscle in your body.

{ 7 }

Just as the movement within the core of your body initiates the abdominal exercise, your inner intentions are manifested in your physical life.

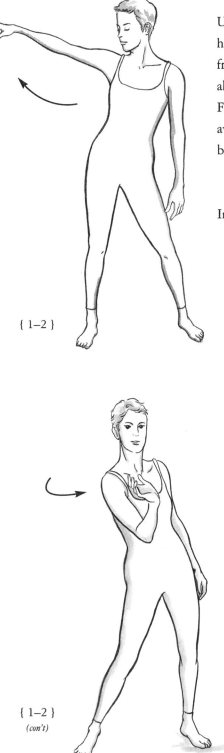

{ 1–2 }

{ 1–2 }
(con't)

Using the same example, we can change our intention by having the movement originate externally rather than from the core. Instead of placing your intention in the abdominal muscle, you can move from the shoulder. Focus on lifting the shoulder off the ground, *then* be aware of the contraction that occurs in the rest of the body once that movement is initiated.

In another example of external movement:

1. Stand facing front with all the joints soft and relaxed. Start moving your right arm by leading with the right hand directly out to the side from the shoulder, then pull it back again.

2. Do this two times, letting the rest of your body follow the movement of the arm. Allow the hips to move *with* the arm back and forth. It's as if the arm and the hips are connected so that the hips and the rest of the body mirror the movement of the arm.

3. Circle the arm out from the hip to the shoulder and across the face and body back to its original position. Do this twice, also letting the hips take on the same circular pattern of the arm.

4. Repeat steps 1, 2, and 3, using the left arm.

There is no right or wrong way for this. The important point is to relax the rest of your body and follow the movement of the arm.

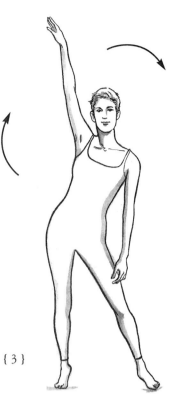

Just as you can let your body follow the motion of your hand, you can relax and "go with the flow," going gracefully with what the universe presents to you.

{ 3 }

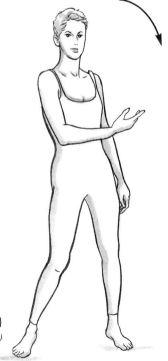

{ 3 }
(con't)

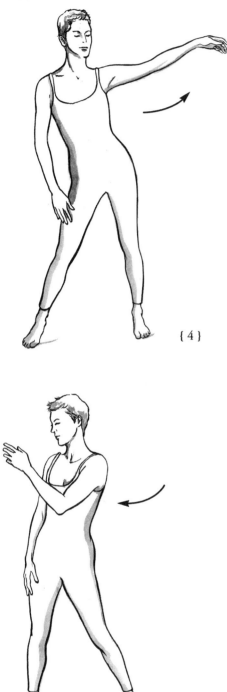

{ 4 }

{ 4 }
(con't)

Reading this metaphor might cause you to wonder, "Why should I go gracefully with something I don't want?" Have you ever railed against something and found that the more violently you resisted it, the more powerfully it came at you? Or if you avoided it in one area of your life, the same thing invariably popped up in another form? Had you gone gracefully with the situation, it would probably have been resolved with a lot less anxiety and pain. This does not mean that you must simply accept everything as it presents itself in life. You should certainly do what you can to release yourself from painful and constricting circumstances, but decrying your fate will only sap the energy that you need to prevail. "Going gracefully" means accepting with equanimity what the universe presents to you; doing so will allow you truly to be in your power and create the reality you want. This is the most efficient use of your chi.

The journey toward balancing your energy and emotions is a process that may take some time. Every time you utilize a Power Practice, you will reinforce this process. Some situations will be harder than others to pull your energy back from, because they are highly charged for you. In some instances, you will find that the process is almost instantaneous. Don't expect to achieve a state of equanimity in all aspects of your life overnight. In fact, let go of all expectations and recognize that you are exactly where you're meant to be. That's really the first step to achieving equanimity. Be gentle with yourself. All of the Power Practices set forth in this book put you on the path to equanimity because they help you to disengage from the fear that keeps you off-balance. Being in your power *is* a state of equanimity.

Your spirit and the universe cocreate your reality. Together, they manifest what you need to learn so that you can evolve. This evolution is a process that occurs one step at a time. Everything that you have experienced has taken you to this point. Even what you might have considered to be "negative" occurrences or setbacks, in fact, served the purpose of helping you learn whatever lessons you needed to learn. Right now you are exactly where you're meant to be, and this is but one step in your journey. You are, at this moment, poised to take the next step forward in your evolution.

Each of the following Chakra Power Practices starts with the following information: Color, Focus, and Points of Power. For each chakra there is then a Short Practice, followed by three levels of exercise to empower your energy centers. Level 1 requires the least physical exertion. Levels 2 and 3 are increasingly aerobic. Keep in mind that since you are working with moving energy, Level 1 can be just as effective as Level 3 in empowering your chakras. Level 3 is simply a more aerobic movement, which involves greater use of your body and augments the free flow of chi. Choose which level you want to do according to how you feel. For each practice, there is also a movement metaphor to connect your physical movement with different aspects of your life. All of the affirmations in this book can be used as the basis of brief, centering meditations to reinforce whichever Power Practice you are utilizing.

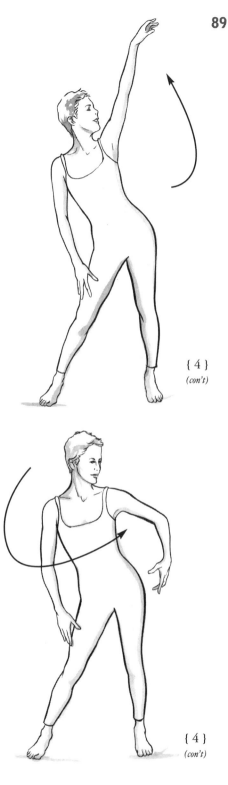

{ 4 }
(con't)

{ 4 }
(con't)

Chapter 12

ROOT CHAKRA

Color: Red

Focus: Roots, Family of Origin, Tribe

Points of Power: Tailbone and Perineum

Many of us had the shakiest of foundations when we were growing up. Part of our journey is learning to keep only what was good and nurturing in our upbringing, while forgiving the rest. We can then form our own foundation, our own tribe. In other words, we can create our own root system of family, friends, and beliefs and build our houses on rock (*yourself, faith, love*), not on sand (*other people, neediness, fear*).

When you base your happiness and emotional security on the behavior or opinions of others, you undermine the foundation of your self-esteem and give away your power. Other people may enhance your life with joy and love, but your sense of self and peace of mind should originate within. You will enrich your life by having loving relationships with others, but you are not an incomplete person who needs to combine with others in order to be whole. You are empowered on your own.

Short Practice

If you feel that you are giving away your power from the root chakra, reclaim your chi by simply unplugging.

To empower you further in this chakra when you are feeling emotionally or physically off-balance, here is an exercise that can ground you at any time, wherever you are.

1. From a sitting or standing position, make sure that your feet are flat on the floor. Keep all of your joints soft (not locked).

2. Press your tailbone downward and reach up through the crown of your head, making your spine very long and relaxed. Notice that you will involuntarily take a deep breath as you create more space in your body.

3. Imagine that you are breathing in beautiful, brilliant, clear energy from the Earth, up through your feet, through your perineum. It courses throughout your entire body.

4. Breathe the light from the heavens down through the crown of your head. Every time you take a breath, you are breathing chi up from the Earth and down from the heavens. As you exhale, see the brilliant light of the energy spread deeper into your body.

5. Take a moment to feel that you are firmly grounded between heaven and Earth. You can now resume whatever you were doing from a more balanced perspective.

Level 1 Exercise

1. Sit on the floor, legs crossed. Feel the light and energy from the Earth entering through the perineum (the space between your pubic bone and your tailbone).

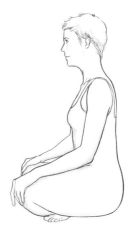

{ 1 }

2. Let the head drop gently toward the chest and let the tailbone tilt upward toward the chin, rounding the spine. (Your body is now in the shape of a **C**.)

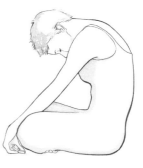

{ 2 }

3. Gently push the tailbone straight down toward the earth. Starting from that small movement, stack each successive vertebra on top of the tailbone, one at a time, as you make the spine very straight.

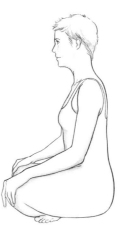

{ 3–4 }

4. Visualize the color red. See in your mind's eye the spacing of the vertebrae as you lengthen the spine. Make sure that your head straightens out last.

 Just as you are lengthening the spine from the initial movement of the tailbone, you grow up into the world from the grounding of your family foundation. Even if your family life was extremely difficult, you learned to survive and are grounding *yourself* through your exploration and discovery of who you really are.

5. Tilt the tailbone toward the back of the head, arching the spine, allowing the head to drop back. Again, straighten the tailbone down toward the Earth and stack the vertebrae, one at a time, straightening the spine.

6. Repeat this exercise until your spine feels relaxed and lengthened. At the same time, visualize the red of the root chakra as it is becoming more clear, radiant, and brilliant.

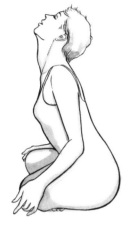

{ 5 }

As your spine flows into orderly movement initiated by the movement of your tailbone, so your life falls into perfect alignment when you are growing from the root of your true self.

Affirmation:
I am safe and grounded. I am building
a solid foundation that allows me to
grow and flourish in the world.

Level 2 Exercise

1. Stand with your feet directly under your hip joints. Imagine that there is a weight on your tailbone, so that it is slightly dropped. Your knees are soft, hips relaxed, feet firmly on the floor. Visualize the color red.

2. Step out with the heel of your right foot; then let the rest of the foot contact the floor, allowing your tailbone to drop even more as you bend your knees out over your toes. Feel the heaviness of the tailbone. Let the pelvis feel loose and buoyant as if it were floating in water.

You can step forward on your path in any direction you choose, balanced and supported by your solid foundation.

3. Pick up your left foot and take a step out in any direction, again leading with the heel, being aware of the balancing effect of your tailbone.

4. Continue with this exercise until you feel balanced and flexible, seeing in your mind's eye the color red, which is becoming clearer and brighter as you open up this energy center.

Affirmation:
My roots fix and stabilize my movement
into the world. I walk forward on my path
deliberately and surely, choosing my own way.

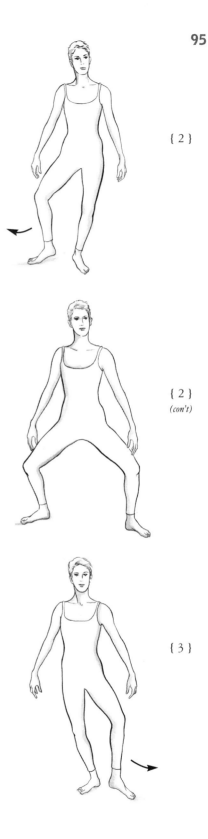

{ 2 }

{ 2 }
(con't)

{ 3 }

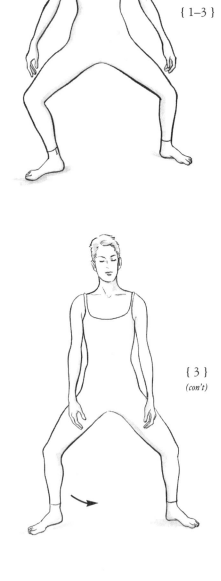

{ 1–3 }

{ 3 }
(con't)

Level 3 Exercise

1. Stand with your feet in a wide stance, more than hip distance apart. Your knees are soft. Feel that your feet are on solid ground, breathing energy up from the Earth through the soles of the feet. Visualize the color red.

2. Gently push the tailbone downward again as if there were a weight tied to it. Then slowly lengthen the spine up through the crown of the head, focusing on the spacing between your vertebrae. (This is a very subtle movement, involving only the tailbone, spine, and head.)

3. Let the tailbone drop more, bending your knees out over the toes. Then, move your right foot next to the left. As you move your feet together, reach up. Your body feels very long as you draw your arms up over your head. When you lift your arms, you are lifting from the rib cage, creating a lot of space between the rib cage and the hips.

4. Step out with your left foot into a wide stance, letting the tailbone drop down, bending your knees as you lower your arms. Move your feet back together by bringing your left foot in, reach up, then step out with the right foot, repeating this exercise until your body feels warm and energized.

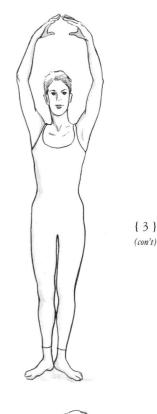

{ 3 }
(con't)

As you lengthen your body more and more, remember that you are able to use your strong, balanced foundation to grow as much as you choose, all the way to your highest consciousness.

Affirmation:
I use the basis of my solid
roots to reach upward to a
higher awareness of my
true self.

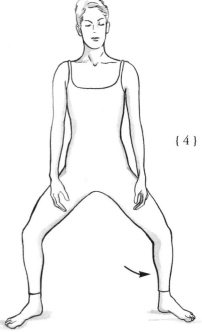

{ 4 }

Meditation and Practice
Root Chakra: Reprogramming Your DNA

Many believe that our DNA carries the blueprint for not only our physical attributes, but also our tendency toward certain behavior patterns. Focusing your energy and intention on changing your behavior at the most basic level of your anatomy will intensify your ability to transform yourself.

1. Lie down in a comfortable position with your spine straight. Take a deep breath and close your eyes. Call your energy, your spirit, your thoughts into this moment. Feel the power of being fully present in this moment.

2. As you relax or get into a meditative state, breathe deeply and become aware of the rhythms of your body. All of the cells in your body have exactly the same DNA. When you change the DNA in one of your cells, the genetic blueprint in every cell changes in exactly the same way.

3. In your mind's eye, see yourself go through a single cell to its center. See the spiral, ladderlike structure of your DNA. As your consciousness is placed in the center of this spiral, ask the universe to assist you in releasing all of the behavior patterns that you learned in childhood that no longer serve you. Send light, love, and energy into your DNA with loving intention.

4. Release these actions and beliefs with gratitude, acknowledging that they helped you to arrive at this moment of healing. You don't even have to know specifically what these actions are. Just ask that they be released.

5. Ask the universe to encode in your DNA healthy, new behavior patterns that will support your continued growth.

Know that your request is heard and acted upon. Remember that the universe *always* hears you, loves you, assists you. You need only ask. Be assured that you are on the right path. Breathe deeply and draw your consciousness back from the cellular level to your larger reality.

Janice's Experience

Janice grew up in a home where both of her parents were active alcoholics. They married when they were seventeen years old because Janice's mother had become pregnant. It is widely believed that alcoholics, unless they enter recovery, never mature past the age when they started drinking. Her parents always acted as if they were in high school, even after they had two other children. Janice and her siblings witnessed their parents' open hostility, drinking, and drugging. This couple was utterly incapable of caring for their children's material or emotional needs. As a young adult, Janice fell into the following pattern. She would become involved with a man and, at first, be very open and available sexually. Then, when Janice was in a relationship that seemed solid and lasting, she put her partner in a position of caretaker. It felt to Janice as though all of a sudden she had lost her physical desire for her boyfriend, although she still loved him. Invariably, Janice avoided sex if she possibly could. In her late teens, Janice began to have cervical and rectal disorders that placed her boyfriend in the role of parent rather than partner. He would take care of Janice without having any sexual expectations, because of her many illnesses.

Her unstable beginnings caused Janice to lose so much chi in her Root Chakra that she didn't have enough energy to keep the area healthy. Janice could greatly benefit from therapy to help her explore her deep wounding around the unavailability of her parents. Chi Fitness would help her ground herself by doing the Root Chakra Exercises and asking herself the Four Questions. She would then be able to explore the roots of her neediness, which stemmed from her experience with her neglectful parents. From this exploration, she could become conscious of why and how she seeks to make other people (such as her boyfriend) into parental figures. By discovering where her energy is leaving her body, she will learn which chakras to focus on when doing Power Practices to reclaim her chi. Through the use of self-talk, she can build a solid foundation of emotional support with *herself* as a base. Additionally, she can add support from friends and therapists who are unconditional in their regard for her.

Chapter 13

EXTERNAL POWER CHAKRA

Color: Orange

Focus: Power in the External World, Creativity

Points of Power: Lower Abdomen and Pelvis

The External Power Chakra has to do with the many ways that we express our power in the world: our careers, relationships, sexuality, and money. This book focuses on the creativity aspect of this energy center, because creativity is necessary to our power. Money comes to us as a direct result of how we express our creativity. In order to have a successful relationship, we must use our creativity to adapt and compromise with others. We use our knowledge in a creative way in order to do our work. In turn, sexuality creates life and the act of sex is a creative use of our bodies.

External power is positive when our intention is to express our inner selves in the outer world lovingly and without fear. External power becomes negative when we seek to have control over others. When you are in a position of power, you can use it in a fear-based or a love-based way. At work and at home, you can be a tyrant—demanding that your children and employees carry out your orders to the letter—or you can be a guide, a positive mentor, and a role model. It is an expression of fear when you can't tolerate another person's individuality. Love is at the root of your behavior when you honor the intelligence and motives of others.

This does not mean that you let your children or employees behave in irresponsible or dangerous ways. It means instead that you direct them, not command them. You can let logical consequences come into play. For the employee, irresponsibility means demotion or termination. For the child, irresponsibility means loss of privileges. Instead of commanding with the energy of fear, you can discipline with the energy of love and kindness.

Many of us are told as children that we cannot be a powerful presence in the world, that power is the right of others more talented and special than we are. We learn the true extent of our power when we use our creative talents, whether in a personal relationship or at work, with the love-based intention "What can I give?" rather than the fear-based thought "What can I get?"

Your creativity and its expression are what make your inner light shine outward. Your power in the world is the direct result of what stems from your creative inner life. The following exercises are designed to help you unblock your creativity, reclaim your chi from power struggles, and strengthen your relationships.

Short Practice

If you feel power loss in this chakra, immediately unplug. To empower yourself further and to unblock this energy center:

1. Start with your feet flat on the floor and press your tailbone downward, lifting up through the crown of the head and straightening the spine. You will automatically take in a deep breath. Visualize the color orange, vibrant and beautiful.

2. Imagine that your pelvis is a balloon. Breathe through the lower abdomen, feeling the balloon expand forward, visualizing the color orange. Exhale, letting the balloon gently deflate.

3. Breathe through the lower back, expanding it, keeping it loose and relaxed. As you breathe in and out, the balloon contracts and expands in both the lower abdomen and the lower back. Breathe this way a few more times, straightening the spine just as you did in the beginning of this exercise.

4. Continue breathing deeply as you return to whatever you were doing, feeling empowered by the flow of chi through this energy center.

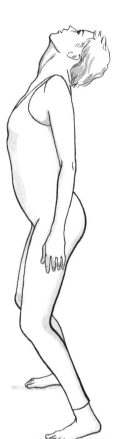

Level 1 Exercise

1. Place your feet in a wide stance, a little more than hip distance apart. The knees are soft, hips relaxed. Start by feeling that there is a weight tied to your tailbone so that it is pointed down.

2. Tilt your pelvis so that your tailbone is moving upward toward the back of your head. Since your pelvis is the point of power in this exercise, let the rest of your body naturally follow its motion. This is a small, subtle movement. Your back will arch slightly and your head can drop back a little.

3. Breathe through your lower abdomen, visualizing the color orange. As you do this exercise, notice that the space between your pubic bone and navel will lengthen, expand, and open while the space in the lower back will shorten, contract, and close.

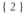 Just as your abdomen expands outward, you let your creativity flow out into the world as a natural extension of your self.

{ 2 }

4. Expand and breathe through the lower back and contract your lower abdomen. Let the rest of your body follow this movement, with your head dropping forward as you pull in the stomach and lengthen the lower back. These movements can be exaggerated by letting your knees get softer and loosening your pelvis even more.

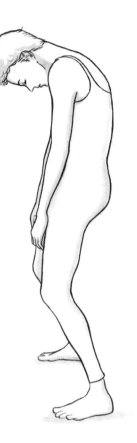

As you contract or close the abdomen, you are "pulling back" physically in the same way you would pull back emotionally if you needed to create a healthy boundary in your job or relationship.

Affirmation:
I can express my power in
the world while also
maintaining healthy
boundaries.

{ 4 }

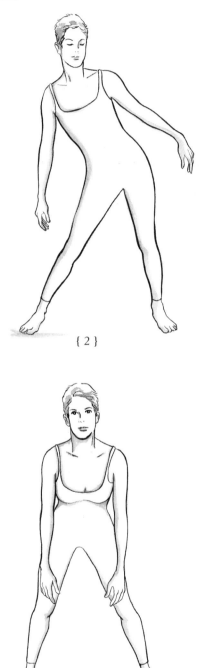

{ 2 }

In the context of external power, creating and maintaining healthy boundaries are essentially the same as staying in your power. They are also a self-esteem issue, which will be discussed in the next chapter. When you are expressing your power in the world, a boundary needs to be maintained that addresses how far you will go with your power. In other words, will you maintain your power or will you relinquish it? Will you allow yourself to be controlled or will you try to dominate others? Your task is to manage your power through love and not fear, inspiring and collaborating with people instead of intimidating or manipulating them.

Level 2 Exercise

1. Start with your feet hip distance apart, tailbone weighted, knees and hips soft and relaxed. Picture the color orange.

2. Rock your pelvis forward and back, then from side to side. Move your hips in a circle, first clockwise, then counterclockwise. Remember to let your hips feel buoyant, as though they are floating in water. Allow your body, not your intellect, to decide which way your pelvis will move.

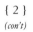 Just as you "let go" and let your body take charge of what movement to do and when to do it, allow your creativity to take its own form and shape.

{ 2 }
(con't)

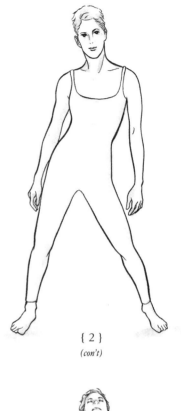

Affirmation:
My power in the world is
a natural extension of my
creativity.

People are often afraid to show others the extent of their creativity. Maybe you are afraid that your skills aren't good enough, that others will think you are showing off, or that your ideas don't fit into what's considered "normal." If you can let go of preconceived notions about what should be and allow your inspirations the light of day, everybody benefits. Let your creativity shine through without stifling it. Even when it's necessary to direct your creativity toward the solution of a specific problem, the concept of "lateral thinking" encourages you to imagine improbable answers, since this can lead to unexpected breakthroughs you might not have otherwise considered. The key is letting go of judgment and self-censorship during this phase of the creative process.

{ 2 }
(con't)

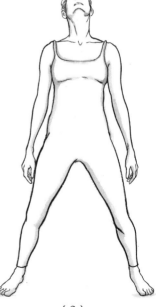

{ 2 }
(con't)

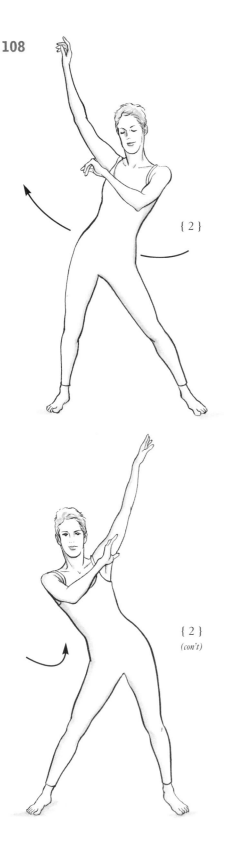

{ 2 }

Level 3 Exercise

1. Stand with your feet hip distance apart. Keep your knees and hips loose and relaxed with your tailbone weighted and pelvis buoyant. Straighten your spine by pushing gently down through the tailbone and reaching up through the crown of the head. Visualize the color orange in your mind's eye, bright and beautiful.

2. Rock the pelvis from side to side and swing your arms to the same rhythm. As the right hip swings to the right, both arms swing toward the right shoulder. Repeat on the left side. Do this exercise for as long as you like.

{ 2 }
(con't)

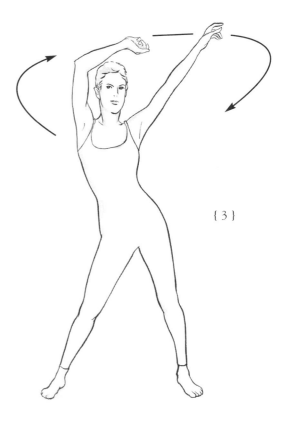

{ 3 }

3. Rotate the pelvis clockwise, circling the arms over the head. Repeat in a counterclockwise motion. Get the feeling that your entire body, including the head, is following the movement of the pelvis.

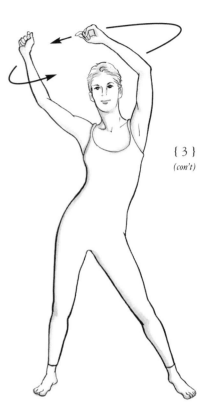

{ 3 }
(con't)

Just as the pelvic movement affects the movement of the rest of your body, the many ways you express your creativity in the world shape your entire life.

If the rest of your body tries to resist the movement of the pelvis, you will feel awkward and could even injure yourself. In the same way, if you try to fight or block the natural expression of your creative nature, the rest of your life won't fall into place.

Affirmation:
My creativity expresses my
power in the world.

Taking your energy back from a power struggle involves combining three of the Basic Power Practices: Power in Present Time, Reclaiming Your Chi, and Spiritual Perspective. It also includes the short practice for your External Power Chakra.

Meditation and Practice
Eliminating Power Struggles

1. Get into a sitting position with the spine straight and relaxed. Breathe deeply and close your eyes. Be aware of the air coming in through your nose as you are infused with brilliant, radiant, healing light. As you breathe, let go of everything that is not here and now. Unplug your energy, your spirit, your thoughts from the past with gratitude for its lessons and gifts and call your chi into this moment. Unplug your energy from your worries for the future, remembering that you are exactly where you're meant to be, trusting that tomorrow takes care of itself. Call your chi from the future into this moment. Continue deep breathing until you feel relaxed, centered, and present.

2. In your mind's eye, visualize the person you're having the power struggle with. The very fact that you are in a power struggle indicates that you are giving your energy away to this person.

3. See whether you can envision your chi leaving your body from your External Power Chakra, between your pubic bone and belly button. You may perceive your energy as leaving you in what looks like a string or cord going from your body to hers.

4. Notice whether the orange color in this chakra seems dull or washed out. Can you sense the chi in this chakra? Does it seem sluggish? It's important not to judge yourself: just take note.

5. Send your energy upward, rising above the mental picture you have of this person, and look down on the entire situation. You now have a larger view of the circumstances surrounding both of you. Looking from this expansive perspective, see whether you can understand what lesson her spirit is playing out for you. Other people's lessons, including hers, don't count here. Only *your* lessons do. If you can't find the lesson, see whether

you can accept that there *is* a larger purpose for these events in your life, whether you understand it or not.

6. Return to where she is right in front of you. Again, see your chi draining from your second chakra to her. Send light, love, and gratitude to this person for whatever her spirit is trying to teach you.

7. Pull these strings of chi out from her energy system, just as if they were electrical cords. Unplug your energy from her and pull it back to you.

8. Visualize the picture of this person as fading until all that is left are light, love, and peace.

9. See the orange color in your External Power Chakra become more bright and alive. Picture the chi in this center as even more vibrant and energetic. Feel the extra boost of power that is now yours.

It is important to remember that unplugging your energy from someone doesn't mean that you are abandoning her or that you don't love her. It means that you are not only regaining your power, but allowing her to be in her power, too.

Keep in mind that it is possible you are losing chi to this person from other chakras in your energy system. For instance, your Voice Chakra could be involved, since this energy center also has to do with your will. If you perceive that this is the case, you can go to the exercises for the Voice Chakra to unblock and empower this center, too.

Short Practice
Eliminating Power Struggles

You can do this the moment you realize you are giving away your chi in a power struggle. Visualize your External Power Chakra and its orange color.

Breathe through this center, pulling back your energy into your lower abdomen and back. Picture the color orange as getting more brilliant as you reclaim your chi.

All of our relationships are in place so that we will learn and grow from them. That is their purpose. Within each of us is the brilliant, perfect light of spirit. What we need to remember is that we all spring from the same perfect source. So deep down, we *are* that perfection. Your present state of being, and that of everybody else, may not seem perfect to you—and it isn't. We're human. But at the core of your being, your soul is perfect and so is everyone else's.

When we first fall in love with our partner, we clearly see his wonderful qualities. We call this stage of the relationship *infatuation.* Time goes by and little things (in fact, the very characteristics we used to adore) start to annoy us. We see his faults. He no longer looks so wonderful. We look back at the infatuation phase, thinking what an illusion it was, what a lie. We now think his flaws are the reality of who he is—but when we saw the perfection and magnificence of our partner, they were the truth. His faults arise from his wounds, not his true self. It is important to remind ourselves not only of our own perfection, but of the perfection of all others as well.

Meditation and Practice
Seeing the Truth in Relationships

1. Get into a sitting position, feet flat on the floor, spine straight. Breathe in brilliant, clear, healing light. Continue to breathe deeply, unplugging your energy, your spirit, your thoughts from everything that is not here and now.

2. See your partner in your mind's eye, sitting directly in front of you. Let yourself think of his shortcomings.

3. Visually place these flaws on the image of his body as little places of darkness. (Accuracy is irrelevant here; only intention counts.)

4. As you are looking at this picture of your partner, with his faults showing on his body, remember that they are not really weaknesses, but *wounds*.

5. Send love and light to this image of your partner, especially to those wounded areas. Look even deeper into this picture, through what appears on the surface.

6. As you look deeper into your partner's true self, his flaws and imperfections dissolve into the light that you are sending him.

7. Once again, recognize the perfection at his core, his dazzling light. Acknowledge that your light is exactly the same as his. Bless him; bless yourself. Whenever you feel ready, open your eyes with this expanded perception of your partner.

Couples' Meditation

1. Sit facing your partner with your spine straight, body relaxed. Close your eyes. Breathe in brilliant, radiant, clear, healing light. Let it enter every cell, dissolving your stress and worries as you draw your chi, thoughts, and spirit into this moment. With every breath you become more radiant and peaceful.

2. Move your attention to your Root Chakra. Visualize brilliant red light. Now, using the intention of your mind, send out some of that beautiful red light toward your partner. Let the energy and color of this energy center meet between your bodies. See in your mind's eye the red, ball-shaped chi of the Root Chakra created by the combination of your energies between you.

3. Raise your attention up to the External Power Chakra between the pubic bone and belly button. Visualize the color orange, brilliant and

vibrant. Send some of the energy and color of this chakra forward to meet your partner's in the middle, creating the second chakra between you.

4. Continue up the body, repeating this exercise all the way up to the seventh chakra.

The Internal Power Chakra is yellow and located in the solar plexus.

The Heart Chakra is green and at the center of the chest.

The Voice Chakra is blue and at the base of the throat.

The Intuition Chakra is at the center of the forehead and is indigo.

The Unity Chakra is purple and located at the crown of the head.

5. As you share and combine your energies in partnership, you create your relationship as an entity. In order for the relationship to thrive, it needs to be supported and nurtured, just as you would nourish, honor, and lovingly care for a beloved child.

6. Remember that you are not giving away your chi in this exercise. You are separate, strong, distinct individuals with particular needs and talents who have chosen to share your lives by creating a relationship.

7. When you feel ready, affirm your commitment to yourself, to the growth of your partner, and to your relationship. Breathe deeply and open your eyes.

A Personal Note

I have always had a lot of trouble exhibiting any power out in the world. Like many women of my generation, I was brought up to believe that I should marry a man who would take care of me, financially and emotionally. The litany in my home was "It's just as easy to fall in love with a rich man as a poor man." I never consciously thought that was true but realized later in life that I did hold the archetype of Cinderella in my psyche. I learned this fact about myself while taking a week-long training intensive with Caroline Myss and Norm Shealy. I was fascinated and chagrined. When I went back to my room that night I prayed for a dream to explain this revelation to me. What I dreamed was hilarious. In it I found a large penis that I sewed to my body. When I finished, I wondered about my female parts. I thought, "Don't worry about it. I can have this penis and still keep my female apparatus, too." Then I looked over and saw Drew standing near me. I realized that I hadn't taken his penis and thought that he would enjoy this transformation as much as I would. For a moment, I was concerned about how to fit this new body part into the front of my pants. Then I said to myself, "Men figure out how to do this all the time. I'll figure it out!"

After I woke up and stopped laughing, I realized the dream's significance. First, I subconsciously felt that to be successful, I had to have a penis—so I found one and put it on. Second, since I didn't take Drew's penis, my success wouldn't emasculate him. In fact, he'd like it. And, third, I didn't have to worry about the mechanics of my newfound appendage. I'd figure it out, just as men do.

That dream changed the energy in my External Power Chakra. I still had work to do, but it completely inspired me. Less than a year later, I made the leap to expand my business, forming a partnership with Drew and moving into a much bigger studio.

Chapter 14

INTERNAL POWER CHAKRA

Color: Yellow

Focus: Self-Esteem

Points of Power: Solar Plexus and Rib Cage

Many of us take quite a beating in the area of self-esteem. We grow up and think, "Who am I that I should have work I love, lots of money, a happy marriage?" The truth is, we love who we love, we enjoy what we enjoy, we want what we want—all for a purpose. We are here to share our gifts, in the workplace, at home, with our friends and families. We all share the same majestic light that lies within. We need to remember who we really are and behave and act accordingly.

Having healthy self-esteem has nothing to do with conceit, which is another form of fear. Paradoxically, it's the fear of not being good enough. When you are conceited, you give the impression that you think you are better than everyone else. Obviously this thought leads to behavior that is not based in love. Conceit is actually an overcompensation for feelings of deep inadequacy. Healthy self-esteem means that you love yourself while also being able to honor other people.

Short Practice

If you have relinquished your chi in this chakra, immediately reclaim it by pulling your energy back to you. To empower your self-esteem further when you find that you are losing your confidence:

1. Place your attention in your solar plexus. Breathe through this area, visualizing the color yellow, brilliant and vibrant.

2. As you breathe in, picture your rib cage as getting bigger, expanding the space between each rib. As you exhale, relax your rib cage to normal size.

3. Continue breathing into this energy center, seeing the yellow light become more vivid and bright. When you have regained your trust in yourself, you can stop the exercise and act with a healthy, reinvigorated sense of self-confidence.

Level 1 Exercise

1. Stand with your feet hip distance apart, with the tailbone pointing straight down as though there were a weight tied to it. Knees are soft and bent directly over the toes. Visualize the color yellow.

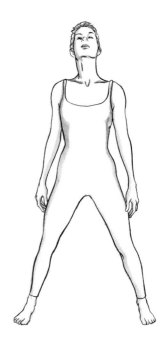

{3}

2. Isolate your rib cage by pretending that from hip to toe, your body is in cement. The upper body is upright, loose, and relaxed.

3. Move only your rib cage. First gently push it forward, then go back to center. Next, push your rib cage backward and return to center.

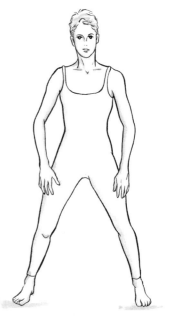

{ 3 }
(con't)

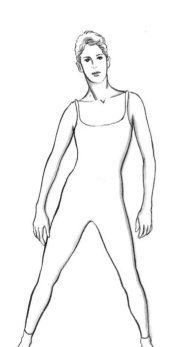

{ 4 }

4. Move the rib cage to the right, still keeping the lower body stationary. Move it to the left. Then move the rib cage in a circular motion—left, forward, right, and backward.

{ 4 }   Just as you move your rib cage from the center of your body, your actions in the world emanate from your core belief that you are worthy, talented, and brilliant.

5. Proceed with this clockwise motion for as long as you like. Then try circling in the other direction. Continue until this energy center feels open and vibrant.

Affirmation:
My self-esteem is the
positive, powerful source
that directs my actions in
the world.

{ 4 }
(con't)

If you are having trouble isolating your rib cage in the exercise, it is probably because you're not used to moving from that point of power. Keep trying. Remember that it's important to maintain a balance between challenging yourself and not pushing too hard. As you practice the movement while placing your awareness in your rib cage, it will loosen up. Visualizing the movement of your rib cage will also be helpful. Awareness and practice are the keys.

Level 2 Exercise

1. Starting with your feet together, tailbone dropped and knees soft, pick up your right foot and step out forcefully to the right while straightening out the right arm in a swift, striking motion directly from the shoulder. Be sure to keep the elbow soft and don't straighten it or "lock" the joint. Stop just short of straightening the elbow completely. Your hand should be palm down, fingers together. As you strike out with the right arm, exhale vocalizing the sound "Huh!" as if you were a martial artist. Feel that you are projecting this sound from the solar plexus.

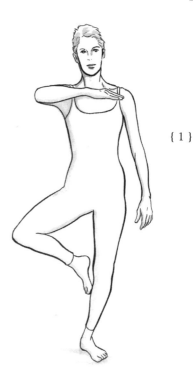

{ 1 }

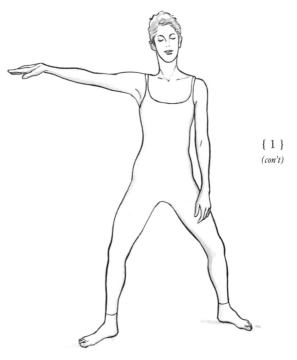

{ 1 }
(con't)

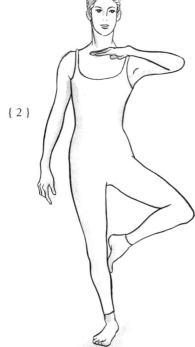

{ 2 }

2. Repeat with your left arm and leg, again vocalizing powerfully from the solar plexus. Visualize the color yellow and continue these movements until you feel powerful and energetic in your Internal Power Chakra.

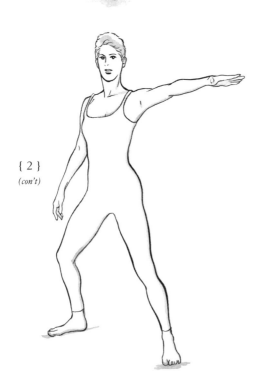

{ 2 }
(con't)

Just as you move and vocalize powerfully from the center of your body, your core strength of healthy, positive self-esteem moves you in the world with confidence and strength.

Affirmation:
I have the confidence and
inner strength to move
powerfully in the world.

Level 3 Exercise

1. Start with your feet about hip distance apart. Cross the right foot over the left, making your whole body face left. Most of your weight should be on the right foot. At the same time, using your rib cage as your point of power, swing your right arm in the same direction as your right foot.

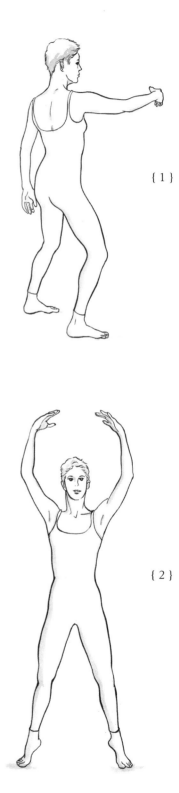

{ 1 }

2. Move your right foot back to center, circling your arms over your head while lifting the rib cage. Make sure the movement upward is from the rib cage and *not* the shoulders. Keep the shoulders relaxed. If you want to make this movement more aerobic, go up on the balls of your feet as you circle the arms over the head.

3. Cross your left foot over the right, letting your body turn toward the right. Most of your weight is now on the left foot. At the same time, keeping your left arm at shoulder height, swing it in the same direction as your left foot, using the motion of the rib cage to move the arm.

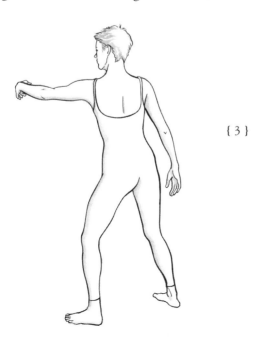

{ 3 }

{ 2 }

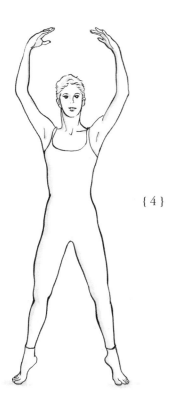

{ 4 }

4. Go back to center, circling the arms overhead. Start again with the right foot and repeat as many times as you like, visualizing the color yellow.

Just as the rib cage motors your arms and causes your body to lengthen at the center position, your joyous sense of self gives you the impetus to move in any direction you wish.

Affirmation:
My actions and behavior
are manifested from the
core belief that my
authentic self is powerful
and can move me to any
place I desire.

You might wonder why, if your soul is perfect, it still needs to evolve. The answer lies in the fact that evolution is a process of linear time. Souls evolve in our physical reality, because we perceive and experience time in this way. In actuality, time is not linear. It simply *is*. This belief has been held by philosophers and mystics for thousands of years and is also a fundamental precept of modern physics. The human experience is that we live our lives from moment to moment and inexorably evolve. This is our perceived reality. But our souls also exist outside this linear realm in an eternal state of perfection, which is, in fact, our true essence. This perfection is always available to us and is manifested when we live our lives in alignment with our souls. Keep this in mind as you practice honoring who you are in the following meditation.

Meditation and Practice
Honoring Who You Are

1. Sit in a comfortable position with your spine straight and relaxed. Call your energy, your spirit, your thoughts into present time. Breathe in brilliant, radiant, clear, healing light. Close your eyes. With every breath you take, you are becoming more radiant, relaxed, and peaceful.

2. Visualize your own brilliant yellow light residing in your solar plexus.

3. As you continue to breathe deeply, see that radiant yellow light shine into every single cell in your body. You are now filled with beautiful, brilliant yellow light.

4. Acknowledge your generous, open, loving heart.

5. Remember that you were created perfect and perfect you remain. Nothing you could ever do or say could make you more perfect; nothing you could ever say or do could make you less perfect. Remember who you are.

6. Acknowledge the brilliance, magnificence, and perfection of your light. Recognize your significance. No one on Earth can achieve what you were sent here to achieve.

7. Acknowledge your power. Every kind thought, every loving gesture emanates from you as healing, yellow light that affects more people than you could ever imagine—just as a pebble thrown into a still lake breaks the surface of the water, with ripples flowing out on all sides, affecting the entire lake.

8. You are perfect, magnificent, brilliant. As you go throughout your day, notice what you say to yourself. Most of us would not be so cruel to our worst enemy. Treat yourself as you would your adored child or dearest friend. Say only loving, encouraging, nurturing words to yourself.

9. Remember and acknowledge the truth of your magnificence. Feel the joy, power, love, and light that are you. Stay in this space for as long as you like. Then, when you feel empowered and relaxed, take a deep breath and open your eyes.

When you lack a certain amount of healthy self-esteem, you tend to have difficulty setting good boundaries. When your limits are blurred, you can actually take on another person's emotions without being aware of it. When you are engaged in a power struggle in a relationship that has poor boundaries, you may actually start to feel the other person's emotions. When you do this, you are basically abandoning yourself. No one in the relationship is then served. By establishing an appropriate boundary, you create the likelihood of a healthier relationship that serves both of you. Creating and maintaining a healthy boundary keep you in your power by making sure you are honoring your own emotions. The following practices show you how to establish and maintain your boundaries energetically in situations that we all encounter.

Short Practice
Creating Boundaries

Suppose you are in conflict with your life partner because you are not happy in your relationship. You are seriously considering separation and you know this information will upset her. Every time you attempt to discuss it, she gets upset. So you back off and never convey what you have to say.

In this scenario, you absorb and actually start to feel *her* feelings, essentially abandoning yourself. Here is a way to change this behavior pattern the next time you talk to her.

Step 1: Use the Basic Power Practice, Power in Present Time.

Step 2: Breathe through your solar plexus, visualizing the color yellow becoming more brilliant and vibrant.

Step 3: Have the intention that this time you will *not* abandon yourself by getting pulled into her feelings. This does not mean that you are not compassionate. It means that you will stay centered in your own emotions. Remind yourself that *nobody* benefits from not knowing the truth.

Step 4: If you start to feel sucked into her panic, take a deep breath and imagine that you are putting a very strong, yet transparent wall between you so that your energy stays on your side and hers stays on the other. Again, remember that you are *not* abandoning her. She gets to own her feelings and to hear your truth; you get to own yours and impart important information to her.

We have all been in situations when we converse with someone and feel as though our energy is being sucked dry. Afterward, we feel exhausted. There are three ways to manage this situation:

1. As described, you can place a wall between your energies.

2. You can place bright, healing, yellow light all around you, with the intention of letting this light transform any energy that passes through it from negative to positive.

3. When you are with someone you find to be energetically draining and you feel negative energy flowing toward you, take it into your body. Send light and love to this energy as though you were comforting a frightened child. Your intention here is to have your love and light transform the

energy from negative to positive. You then send it back to the other person with love and compassion. (*This is the most love-based expression of this practice. Use it at a time when you feel strong and grounded.*)

David's Experience

This example from David's life is illustrative of how children, especially kids who seem "brave" or mature for their years, sometimes feel overly responsible for the events in their households.

Before he learned how to meditate and practice Chi Fitness, David probably lost more energy through the Internal Power Chakra than any other. All of his fear-based emotions were fueled by self-doubt, even when he exuded self-confidence to the outside world. Growing up, he cast himself in the role of first-born family "hero," attempting to negotiate peace in his household—and failing miserably on a daily basis. This feeling of helplessness wormed its way into his self-image and formed an emotional block that persisted into adulthood.

When he explored this chakra with the Basic Power Practices, two incidents, in particular, still held the greatest "charge." The first occurred when he was five years old. His brother was almost two—a playful, adventurous little boy with a halo of blond curls rising from his head. But deep down, David's love for him was tinged with jealousy. Before he was born, David had been the center of his parents' attention. Even if that attention was a double-edged sword, offering both protective love and intimidation, he was still unrivaled for their affection. Now his brother needed their devotion, too. David doubts he was ever aware of these feelings, but something happened that suddenly made his little brother the focus of everyone's concern. David was in his room when he heard his mother scream. His father raced over from the other end of the house. David followed him into his parents' second floor bedroom. Somehow, his brother had climbed up onto the dresser beneath an open window and had fallen out, tumbling onto the bushes below. With his mother in hysterics, David's father called an ambulance and cradled the little boy's inert body until the paramedics sped him away. David wept and clung to his mother, nauseous with terror, feeling helpless and somehow responsible.

His brother miraculously survived the fall and fully recovered, but a sense of guilt and impotence burrowed deeper into David's psyche. Had he wanted him to die? Was it his fault he almost did? These questions hadn't even occurred to David until he asked himself the Four Questions and meditated on this chakra. Until then, every fear-based thought and emotion he experienced was plugged into this incident, sapping energy and undermining his self-image.

Two decades later, another horrific event provoked a similar reaction. David's daughter almost died at birth, and his fear rose up in helpless rage. Despite a very difficult pregnancy, his wife went into labor determined to have the baby "naturally." She and David had enjoyed taking birthing classes together. He was a well-trained, eager "coach" and she was as positive as an anxious first-time mother could be. Labor, though, went on for almost twenty hours and the baby's heart rate suddenly started to plummet. Instead of a well-planned, drug-free process, there was now an emergency. A spinal block had to be injected while his wife was in the middle of a contraction, and the baby was turned and yanked out with forceps. She was blue and motionless but clung to life. After a week in an incubator, she was able to be taken home. But the horrific helplessness David felt, watching his wife suffer and his daughter enter the world so stressfully, was fueled by the same fearful self-reproach. Even while his heart was bursting, it was his solar plexus that felt on fire. The energetic connection of fear to this chakra persisted from childhood. Decades more would pass before David recognized and dealt with it. Although he has done much healing in this area, David's knee-jerk reaction can still be to rescue everyone he loves. When he is reminded of this, he can use a power practice and back off, because once his Internal Power Chakra is energized, he no longer feels the need to save everyone.

Chapter 15

HEART CHAKRA

Color: Green

Focus: Love and Compassion

Points of Power: Center of the Chest and between

the Shoulder Blades

As you already know, there are only two basic emotions from which all others flow: love and fear. When we are angry, judgmental, or envious, we are really afraid. In that moment, we are not loving. When we can recognize that our negative emotions stem from fear, we can use this awareness as a tool for self-discovery to find the roots of our anxiety. These roots are where we've been wounded.

It is essential to acknowledge and feel our fearful thoughts and emotions rather than denying and suppressing them. This is where we have the opportunity to practice love and compassion for ourselves.

The fact of being human makes it necessary to experience and claim all of our emotions authentically.

When we accomplish this, we can feel compassion when other people are behaving in ways that are fear-based. Loving, accepting, and forgiving ourselves pave the way for us to give those same gifts to the other people in our lives.

When you unplug your energy from someone in order to forgive, you take your power back. If you have really forgiven someone, then you are not judging, and you have truly let go of your fear. This is the first level of forgiveness. On the second level you can empathize with the person and feel compassion. Since this is a love-based intention, it further empowers you. The third and most powerful level of forgiveness occurs when you can feel gratitude for the lesson this person gave you. This is not only a love-based perception, but one that reflects the higher awareness of your spiritual nature.

Short Practice

Unplug as soon as you realize that you have given your chi away from your heart center. Empower your heart center further when you are feeling angry, fearful, or judgmental by recognizing that the root of these emotions is fear.

1. Breathe into your heart center, in the middle of the chest, visualizing the color green. As you breathe in, expand the front of your chest so that the heart is opening outward. At the same time, close your shoulder blades by contracting the space between them.

2. As you exhale, open up the shoulder blades, opening the heart center toward the back. At the same time contract your chest.

3. Keep opening and closing the front of your chest and your back, picturing the color green growing brighter and more vibrant. When your heart center feels empowered, resume whatever you were doing with the energy of an open heart.

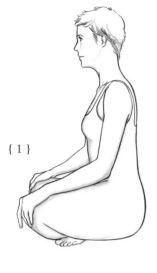

{ 1 }

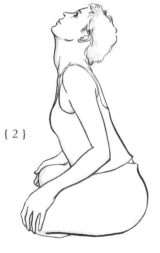

{ 2 }

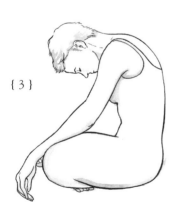

{ 3 }

Level 1 Exercise

1. Get into a sitting position. Lift up through the crown of the head and gently press down through the tailbone, lengthening the spine. Relax into that length.

2. Just as in the Short Practice, inhale and exhale, opening and closing the chest and the shoulder blades. As you breathe in, expand the chest. Bring the shoulder blades together, allowing the head naturally to fall back as you expand the heart center forward. Imagine the color green. Allow your shoulders to stay relaxed as you gently press the shoulder blades together. Leading with the center of the chest, the rest of your body moves from that point of power.

3. Exhale, open up the shoulder blades, and close up the chest, letting the head naturally fall forward, opening the heart center from the back of the body.

Just as you expand the heart center forward with the rest of your body following that point of power, when you "lead" and take action with the intention of love, the rest of your life falls into place with natural ease and harmony.

Affirmation:
I take action in my life according to the wisdom of my heart, knowing that this creates a natural order and harmony.

Level 2 Exercise

1. Take a wide stance with a long, relaxed spine, soft knees, and weighted tailbone.

2. Breathe in, expanding the center of the chest forward while contracting between the shoulder blades, allowing your arms to reach back. Your head will naturally drop back, opening the chest even more.

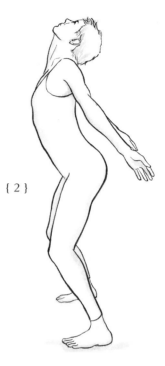

{ 2 }

3. Exhale, opening the space between the shoulder blades, contracting the center of the chest. Keep the shoulders relaxed and allow your arms to move forward. Your head will naturally drop forward. In your mind's eye, see the color green and imagine your energy flowing unhindered through the heart center. Keep doing this until your Heart Chakra feels open and vibrant.

Just as the expansion and contraction of the Heart Chakra expand your body outward and control the movement of the head, you can let go of the intellect and trust the energy of the heart in making decisions as you move forward in your life.

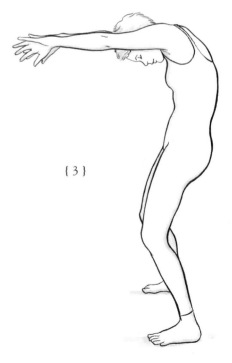

{ 3 }

Affirmation:
I let go of fearful thoughts.
I am empowered by the
energies of love and
compassion.

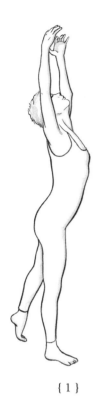

{ 1 }

Level 3 Exercise

1. Start with your feet in a wide stance, tailbone weighted, knees soft. With the right foot, move toward the left by crossing the right foot over the left and letting the whole body face left. Most of your weight is on the right foot. As you cross the right foot over the left, lengthen the spine and expand the center of the chest upward as you circle both arms over the head. See the color green in your mind's eye.

2. Move the right foot back into a stance with the arms straight out from the shoulders, letting the tailbone drop and knees bend out over the toes. Feel the stretch across your chest.

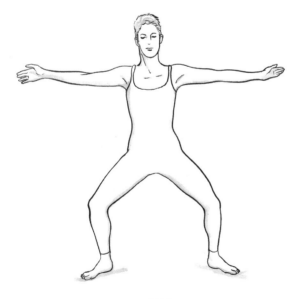

{ 2 }

3. Repeat on the other side, this time crossing the left foot over the right and facing the right side. As you step to the right, lengthen the spine, expanding the heart center with your arms circling over the head.

🌀 Just as you lengthen the spine and expand the heart center upward and outward, you grow up and expand into the richness of your life through the energies of love and compassion.

4. Repeat this exercise. Feel that your spine is lengthening and your chest is expanding more and more each time.

🌀 Just as your chest expands in this exercise, your capacity to embody love and compassion is amplified as you grow from your heart.

Continue with this exercise until you feel that your Heart Chakra is energized and open.

Affirmation:
My spirit soars as I follow my heart.

{ 3 }

It's not unusual to wonder why you should forgive someone who did something awful to you. Most of us are reluctant to forgive because in some way we feel it is letting that person "off the hook." The reality is that when you forgive someone, you are letting *yourself* off the hook. After all, you are not making him suffer by not forgiving him. Honestly, what does he care? You are suffering because you cannot let go of the incident that plagues you.

If there is something in the past that you cannot forgive, you are still plugged into it. When you think of it you feel a charge, a rush of feeling such as anger or shame. This is an indication that you are still relinquishing your chi to this person. In your mind, you go back to the incident repeatedly, expending your chi. The more you hold on to old injustices and pain, the more energy you give to the past. This leaves less chi available for you to use as fuel for your physical, emotional, and spiritual health. Caroline Myss says in her *Energy Anatomy* tapes that *forgiveness is the single best thing you can do for your biology.* When you forgive, the rush of chi into your system provides immeasurable relief to your body and soul.

You may think that you can reclaim your chi simply by having the intention of never again seeing or thinking of the person who has wronged you, but this itself requires energy that is fear-based. You have given your chi away to fearful thoughts rather than empowering yourself with love and compassion. Forgiveness expresses compassion for yourself as well, freeing you from the bondage of fear, blame, and judgment. Be kind to yourself during this process. It is difficult and painful for everyone, and one of the hardest lessons to learn. In the end, the act of forgiveness is really about healing yourself.

This doesn't mean you have to let a toxic person back into your life. Once you have taken care of yourself by practicing forgiveness, you can stay in your power by setting healthy limits concerning what you will and will not accept.

Whenever we can't let go of our anger, whenever we blame someone else, or when we can't forgive, we become ill and bitter, robbing our body and spirit of the energy that keeps us healthy and happy. We drain our heart center of its chi, making it difficult to practice love and compassion. When we forgive, we let go of our fear, healing and energizing the heart center.

The following practice is a combination of the Basic Power Practices: Power In Present Time, Claiming Your Chi, and Spiritual Perception. Forgiveness is one of the *most* important practices. Forgiving does not mean condoning someone else's actions. It means no longer giving your chi away to this incident or person. You empower yourself by letting go of painful memories.

Meditation and Practice
Forgiveness

1. Sit with your spine straight. Lift up through the crown of the head and push down through the tailbone. Take a deep breath; close your eyes. With every breath you take, you are breathing in brilliant, radiant, clear, healing light. It is streaming into every cell of your body. With every breath you take, the light circulates deeper and deeper into your body, dissolving the everyday cares and worries of this life, relaxing you more and more. As you breathe, let go of everything that is not here and now. Unplug your energy, your spirit, your thoughts from the past with gratitude for its lessons and gifts and call your chi into this moment. Unplug your energy from your worries for the future, remembering that you are exactly where you're meant to be, trusting that tomorrow will take care of itself. Call your chi from the future into the present moment. Continue with your deep breathing until you feel relaxed, centered, and present.

2. Make a mental picture of the person you need to forgive. As you are looking at this person in your mind's eye, allow yourself to feel your rage, sadness, hatred, or whatever emotion comes up for you.

3. Be aware that you are giving away your power to this person. See the energy strings leaving your body directly from your heart center and hooking into her energy system.

4. Look at the color green in your heart center. Is it dull? Does the energy in your heart center seem stagnant when you think of this person?

5. In this moment, be aware of three things:

- We all originated from and share the same source. You and this person are connected at the deepest level.

- Before the two of you incarnated into physical form, your spirits agreed that she would demonstrate a great lesson for you. The souls who love us the most agree to teach us the most intense lessons here on Earth.

- When someone does a terrible thing, that person is acting from extreme fear. Can you see that in her?

6. Look at her in your mind's eye. See the green color and the chi in your Heart Chakra. See whether you can pull your chi strings out of this person and back into your heart center. Feel your power return to you in this moment.

7. Look at her and realize that she was acting from fear. Remember when you yourself have acted from fear. See whether you can recall your own terror. As you allow yourself to empathize with this person, see the color and the energy in your heart center get brighter.

8. Project your chi up over your head so that now you see this person and the entire situation that surrounded the two of you when you had this experience together.

9. From this perspective, where you have an even clearer view of events, see whether you can feel compassion for this person. When you allow yourself to feel compassion, your heart center lights up with an even brighter green.

10. Lift your energy even higher and see whether you can feel gratitude for the lesson this person gave you. In this moment, feel the burst of power that moves through your body and energetic system. The energy in your heart center is now a brilliant green. You have fully unplugged your chi, empowering yourself and renewing your physique with vibrant health.

11. Send love to this person as her image fades into the light. Experience the joy and peace that come from forgiving. When you are ready, open your eyes, feeling rejuvenated and energized.

It is important to remember that you do not have to embrace any of the spiritual beliefs set forth in this book to benefit from Chi Fitness. As we've said before, you can do the practices to open up your energy system without having to intellectualize what you are doing. You can simply use the exercises to get the chi flowing freely throughout your body and manage it in your daily life. This will be, in itself, enormously helpful to you.

It is sometimes asking a lot to face looking at old hurts in order to practice forgiveness. You may not feel ready to let go. Don't fool yourself by denying your true feelings. It's wonderful when we can actually feel compassion for those who've wronged us, but it's a difficult task. If you can't bring yourself to feel compassion for a certain person yet, be kind to yourself, admit your authentic feelings, and accept that there are some places on your path to healing that you are not yet ready to explore. When you acknowledge your limits, it is much easier to work through them and progress.

In the forgiveness meditation and practice, the idea is put forth that your soul incarnates into physical form in order to evolve by experiencing situations that cause it to learn and grow. Before physical incarnation, each of us agrees to assist others in their evolution by presenting and participating in certain lessons. Sometimes people who cause our deepest issues to surface are our greatest teachers because they bring about the most profound, life-changing experiences.

We all originate from the same source and remain energetically connected.

So when we send healing energy to somebody who is physically far away from us, he can benefit from it. When you are in a close relationship with another person, the shifts in your energy system cause shifts in hers as well. Here is an everyday example. Say you are having power struggles with your teenage daughter. You want her to dress a certain way, because you *know* what's appropriate. Now suppose you pull your energy out of this conflict and decide to let her wear what she wants. In essence, you have reclaimed your chi and allowed your daughter to own hers. Even if you don't say a word about your decision, your energy has changed. You will find that your daughter's energy has also changed in regard to the situation. She may be less hostile because she can feel that you have let go, so that her reactions are not as extreme as they might have been otherwise. Changing your energy alters your perception and your behavior and affects everyone around you as well. When you forgive or do any practice that empowers you, everyone benefits.

Remember the expression "What goes around comes around"? This means that what you send out to another person you ultimately receive back in some form from the universe. This is commonly thought of as some kind of cosmic revenge or reward system: do something good and something good happens to you; do something bad and you will ultimately suffer. This saying makes more sense if you consider that *we are all one*. It then becomes clear that what you give to someone else, you are also giving to yourself, because we are, in reality, the same being. Therefore, when you send love and light to another, you are also receiving it.

Even if you have mixed feelings about a person, if your intention is to send love, that's what he receives. It's always empowering to send love, whether or not you have some unresolved, fear-based issues regarding him. If this is underlying your relationship, it may well weaken the intensity of your loving intention, but as long as the other person is in *his* power, your fear won't hurt him. When you give away your power in fear, you are the one hurt by it. Furthermore, the practice of Chi Fitness will inevitably unearth your authentic feelings, because your energy system reflects your true emotions. As you become more sensitive to your energetic relationship to this particular person, any underlying emotional and psychological conflicts will be clearer to you. Then you will be able to deal with them more directly.

When you send light and energy to another person with the intention of assisting her with the energy of love, it is *not* the same as giving your power away, because that is unintentional. When you give your chi away, you are experiencing fear in some form. Although losses in your energy system will ultimately weaken you, there is nothing debilitating about intentionally sending out your chi to deliver love and healing to another person. When you project healing energy to someone, it empowers you both.

Short Practice
Compassion

The moment you judge someone else's behavior, realize what you are doing. Then remind yourself that we are all one and the same. We embody the identical light. Recognize the divinity that we all share, including the individual you are judging. Finally, remember that when an individual acts in an unloving way, he does so because he is afraid. His fear has overcome him. Try to stay with this altered perception of him until you begin to feel compassion instead of judgment. Then, from this new perspective, open your heart and send love to help him banish his fear.

This does *not* mean that you need to become this person's doormat. If you are in a situation in which you need to respond to his provocative behavior, this practice helps you respond with love and compassion instead of fear and aggression.

This technique can also be used to help those who are going through a difficult passage such as illness or emotional distress. You can send healing light no matter how far apart you may be physically. Energy transcends space and time. Take a deep breath and picture a loved one in your mind's eye. Send light, love, and energy to him directly from your heart center. When you do this with a healing intention, you will also empower yourself.

A Personal Note

Before my mother died, she was in and out of a hospital in my childhood hometown, Pittsburgh, Pennsylvania. I would fly back and forth for long weekends to be with her. Our friend Karen took over my classes here in Westport, Connecticut. (I am blessed by the good-heartedness of my clients, teachers, and friends.) I remember so clearly one day sitting in my mother's hospital room and feeling love and energy wash over me. I recognized many of my friends' and clients' chi. Looking at the clock, I realized that the Chi Dance class in Westport was ending at that very moment. Karen was guiding the meditation and I could feel that the whole class was sending me light and love. It was powerful energy, incredibly helpful and nurturing to me during that difficult time.

Steven's Experience

The exercises and meditation practices for this chakra helped Steven to heal the deepest emotional wound he experienced as an adult: the end of his marriage. Steven and his wife had known each other since nursery school. The greatest thrill of his life (before the age of twelve) occurred when she held hands with him for the first time as they walked home from school. It was the first time he fell in love. Steven ended up going to a different high school and college, so they didn't spend much time dating until their early twenties, but by the time they got married, their happiness seemed as if it had been destined all along. Steven and his wife both pursued creative careers, parented three wonderful children, and weathered the disappointments of frustrated ambitions with fortitude and mutual support. Over time, though, fear-based anxiety and antagonism began to corrode their relationship. Eventually, it ended in a tailspin of betrayal when she became involved with another man. Steven sank into a state of depression. He kept himself afloat by his devotion to his children, his friends, and whatever creative work he could produce, but his heart felt literally broken. The pain lingered for years, leeching his energy, drawing on all the traumas that had ever poisoned his self-image. Much angst could have been averted had he understood then what he realizes now. His experience, however heartbreaking, was really a catalyst to reveal and heal the wounds that had inhibited his emotional and spiritual growth. The Power Practices, especially those for the Heart Chakra, have enabled him to unplug from any lingering fear-based emotions in his relationship with his former wife, and that in turn empowers him to be fully present in the sacred partnership he happily shares with the woman in his life now. As a result, Steven feels energized with love and gratitude because he understands that everything in his life is created for the evolution of his soul.

Chapter 16

VOICE CHAKRA

Color: Blue

Focus: Voice and Will

Point of Power: Neck

Have you ever had the experience of trying very hard not to cry? You shove the tears way down your throat until it hurts. It can feel as if you are choking. We can all relate to the experience of not being able to express our truth. Feeling it's not permissible to ask for what we want, we hide our true emotions.

On the other hand, asserting your will is an expression of being in your power. This is different from trying to exert control over another person. You can assert your will without being invested in how others react to you. You can speak your truth without trying to control others.

In the following exercises, you will contract and expand the area of the Voice Chakra. (As always, using your thoughts and intentions will intensify this process.) The idea of constricting the neck area originates in healing arts practices, such as yoga and shiatsu, that physically block the flow of chi along an energy meridian, using various techniques to clear, balance, and reinvigorate the energy system. By opening up the Voice Chakra, you can unblock the energy there to exercise your voice and make your will known.

Short Practice

The moment you realize that you are having a hard time speaking your truth or asserting your will, recognize that you have given away your power. Immediately call your energy back, unplugging from the situation or people who are present.

1. Take deep, full, long breaths. Continue to breathe deeply, imagining that you are inhaling clear, radiant energy up from the Earth through the soles of your feet. The energy ascends through all of your chakras to the throat area, then is exhaled through your mouth. Visualize the color blue. As you breathe, picture your throat opening so that chi flows effortlessly through this energy center and the color blue becomes more alive and vibrant.

2. Breathe beautiful, bright energy through the crown of the head downward through the throat, again exhaling through the mouth. When you are feeling empowered in your Voice Chakra, take any opportunity you can to say what is important for you to say.

Level 1 Exercise

1. Sit in a comfortable position with your spine straight. Lift up through the crown of the head and push gently downward through the tailbone. Take a deep breath. See in your mind's eye the color blue.

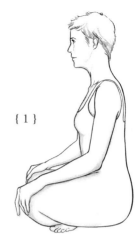

{ 1 }

2. Placing your attention at the front of the neck, inhale and expand this area by allowing the head to drop back and the chest to move slightly forward. To do this, visualize the front of your neck, picturing it as getting bigger as you drop your head back. Moving from this point of power opens up and energizes the Voice Chakra. Visualizing helps you focus your energy and intention. The same technique is used when you expand the back of the neck.

{ 2 }

3. Picture the back of the neck getting bigger and opening up as you exhale. Drop your head forward, allowing the back of the neck to expand and opening the space between the shoulder blades.

Just as the motion of the head and the chest allows the expanded movement of the neck, your voice shows the outside world the truth of your mind and heart.

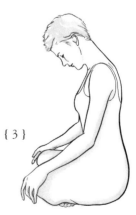

{ 3 }

Affirmation:
I speak the truth of my mind and heart.

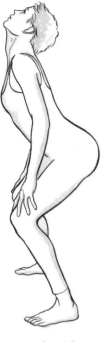

{ 1–2 }

Level 2 Exercise

1. Stand with your feet a little more than hip distance apart, toes pointing forward. Place your hands on the front of your thighs, then sink, bending the knees and arching the back. See the color blue in your mind's eye.

2. Lower your body and open up the chest and neck, dropping your head back. Continue to sink lower until you can't keep your back arched any longer.

3. Allow your head to drop forward, and let it hang, lifting the tailbone up.

Just as the balance between your chest and head keeps the neck open, your voice and will reflect the perfect balance of the wisdom of the heart and the insight of the mind.

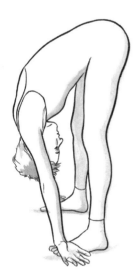

{ 3–4 }

4. You are now in a hanging stretch, legs straight, knees soft. If the stretch in the back of your legs is too intense, bend the knees a little more. Relax and breathe deeply as you hang, feeling lengthening of the spine and stretching in the back of the legs.

5. Keeping the knees soft, push the feet into the floor and slowly straighten up, one vertebra at a time, letting the head go up last.

Affirmation:
The knowledge and desires
of both my mind and my
heart are integrated in the
words I speak.

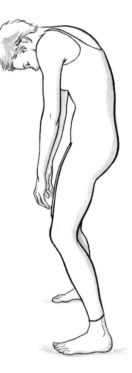

{ 5 }

Level 3 Exercise

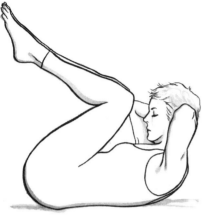

{ 1–2 }

Imagine that you are bending a garden hose that is filling up with water. The water will build up where the hose is bent. It is "blocked." When you unbend the hose, the water rushes through easily and unimpeded. The water is analogous to your chi. When you physically block the area where energy flows, the chi builds up. When you release the block, energy will rush through.

1. Lie down on your back and draw the knees up into your chest. Place your hands behind your head as if you were going to do a sit-up.

2. *Gently* press the chin down toward your chest, expanding the back of your neck while contracting the front of it. Make sure you don't pull on the head with your hands. Your hands are merely supporting your head as you press your chin downward, constricting the front of your throat. Breathe through your nose.

3. Stay in this position for about ten seconds, visualizing the color blue.

4. Slowly uncurl from this position, lowering the head and hips onto the floor.

{ 5 }

5. Get on your knees and sit on your heels, keeping your spine straight. Now lean back, extending your hands back behind the feet, pressing your palms into the floor. Slowly drop your head back, letting your

hands support you. Open up the front of your neck, breathing through your nose and visualizing the color blue. Relax and feel the energy of the Voice Chakra flowing freely.

In this exercise you constrict the energy of the Voice Chakra between the chest and the head. When you release it, your chi flows freely and powerfully through the voice center. In your life, before you use your voice, allow yourself time to balance the energies of the head and heart. Then you can speak your truth powerfully and clearly.

Affirmation:
Before I speak, I pause to listen carefully to my
innermost truth.

Using your voice in meditation (called *sounding*) opens up the Voice Chakra. It also quiets the brain and promotes healing, drawing your body and energy system into a natural state of harmony and balance.

For thousands of years, it has been known that the chanting or "toning" of certain sounds helps to quiet the mind, so that a person can enter a meditative state and achieve deep relaxation. This reduction of stress, in itself, enhances the flow of chi, allowing the body to function better and heal more readily. In *Sounds of Healing,* Dr. Mitchell Gaynor points out that recent research in the field of neuroacoustics provides scientific evidence of how particular sounds resonate within our bodies to promote recovery from illness. These sounds actually stimulate the immune system to produce healing agents and draw the vibrations of our atomic structure into harmonic balance with the universe.

If there are two string instruments in the same room, playing a note on one will cause the other to produce the same sound, even though no one is touching it. The same kind of thing will happen to two metronomes: even though they start with different beats, eventually, of their own accord, the rhythm of their beating will become synchronous. There is a natural state of balance, a vibrational harmony that resonates in every cell of your body and throughout the universe. This may well be why many people have had the experience of hearing a universal harmony in response to their own toning.

Meditation and Practice
Sounding

1. Sit with your spine straight. Lift up through the crown of the head and press down through the tailbone. Take in a deep breath and exhale. Continue to take deep breaths and close your eyes.

2. When you are ready, breathe in, and on the exhale, say, "OHHHHH." Then, as you run out of air, finish with "mmmmmmm" to sound the word *ohm*. Repeat this in the next breath. You can continue with *ohm* or any peaceful sounds you want, allowing your intuition to guide you. Use sounds such as "ahh," "eeee," "aaa," or "mmm."

3. Allow the vibration of your sounds to draw your mind into silence. Let yourself stay in meditation for as long as you like. When you are ready, take a deep breath and open your eyes, feeling renewed and serene.

Clearing the mind is difficult for anyone practicing meditation. The more you want to stop thinking, the more thoughts seem to come to you. When thoughts continue to disturb you, instead of fighting them off, let them enter your mind, but have the intention of not getting pulled into any emotion about them. Look at these thoughts with as much detachment as possible. Eventually, your thoughts will stop. The important thing is to make sure that you don't get upset with yourself. Clearing the mind is a *practice*. And that's exactly what it takes. You also might try to continue sounding without thinking about when you have to stop. Disengaging your mind from what you are doing will allow you to enter a deeper meditative state.

Your body, mind, and energy system are inseparable. The body is animated by chi and contains an intelligence of its own. It repairs itself, follows a genetic blueprint, replaces old cells, and can create new life. However, this intelligence extends beyond the scope of the merely physical. In the following practice, you are letting go of your intellect in order to make a decision in another way. Sometimes, for example, the intellect can fool you into thinking that what is best for you is what makes you the most money, but intellect does not always lead us to joy. Using your chi and your body as decision-making tools gives you an entirely new perspective that can break through patterns of thinking that don't serve you. Making decisions, of course, involves the use of your voice and will. This practice centers on total body chi.

The intelligence of the body and your energy system work together perfectly. As you practice Chi Fitness, you will become increasingly aware of your chi through your bodily sensations. In the Making Decisions Practice, you will receive guidance by interpreting how the energy feels in your body.

Meditation and Practice
Making Decisions

1. Get into a sitting position, spine straight, and take a deep breath.

2. You can sound, focus on your breathing, or do whatever you need to do to quiet your mind.

3. When you feel peaceful and clear, think about the decision that you need to make. Think specifically about what will happen when you make that choice. For example, "I'll take this new job." Notice how your body

feels when you make that statement to yourself. Visualize yourself in that working environment. If your body feels light and unencumbered, your energy system is saying yes. Alternatively, if your body begins to feel heavy and sluggish, the message your body is sending you is no. Trust the intelligence of your body. Your intellect can lie to you; your body won't.

Marty's Experience

Marty was married for seven years to a woman who seemed incapable of intimacy. He was very unhappy and lonely in this relationship. He wanted to avoid divorce, if possible, so he and his wife went into therapy. It became apparent after a few months that therapy was not helping. Their marriage continued to deteriorate. Marty found that he was thinking more and more about separation and divorce. His wife was adamantly opposed, so they kept trying to improve their relationship, to no avail. Marty was torn. He didn't want to hurt his wife, yet he was incredibly unhappy. While Marty was trying to decide what to do next, he noticed that every time he thought about leaving the marriage, his body would feel elated and light as a feather. When he admonished himself, that he'd better stay and continue to try, his body felt so much like a dead weight that he could barely stand up. The difference in Marty's body between yes and no was really that dramatic. Finally, Marty and his wife did get a divorce and they both eventually found other partners. Ultimately, divorce was the best choice for this couple. Marty considers the experience to be an enormous lesson regarding decision making. Now he always listens intently to what his body is telling him.

Since the Voice Chakra is related to will, when an individual has a serious addiction, this chakra will be blocked. The addict attaches his energy to a substance or behavior pattern that actually controls him. Even if you are not an addict, you may still give away your power to substances such as food. You may have a difficult time staying away from foods you should avoid or to the behavior pattern of overeating. Please note that the following practice is not meant to provide a remedy for addiction. For that, an individual needs extensive therapy. However, along with therapy, these exercises may serve to assist you in taking back your power from harmful substances and behavior.

The following exercise is a Short Practice to disengage from substances to which you are relinquishing your power. You've probably had the experience of not being able to control your eating habits when you are trying to lose weight or stay away from foods that cause you to have an allergic reaction. Reclaiming your chi from a substance is the same as unplugging from a person or a situation.

Short Practice
Unplugging from a Substance

Suppose you are trying to diet and you want a chocolate chip cookie. You know that once you have one cookie, you will "crack" and eat at least twelve. To take your power back, simply take a deep breath and visualize the energy cord running from your throat right into that cookie. Then pull the plug out of the cookie back into your throat area, picturing the color blue as becoming more radiant and clear as you reclaim your chi.

Once you call your energy back, do the Short Practice for the Voice Chakra. When you cannot let go of unhealthy eating habits, it's really a form of punishing yourself. Therefore, you might also want to look at your self-esteem energy center and energize that chakra by performing some of those exercises. You can also visualize your body exactly as you want it to be, knowing that this will be a powerful tool for change.

Chapter 17

THE INTUITION CHAKRA

Color: Indigo

Focus: Intuition and Power of the Mind

Point of Power: Forehead

In most cultures today, we are brought up to discount and even distrust our intuition. Even for people of profound religious faith, the world of instinct and feeling isn't concrete enough to verify or validate in everyday life. Children trust their instincts until they are taught otherwise. Remember when you could *see* that a person was saying all the right things, but you *felt* he was deceitful? Probably your first impressions were accurate. We are taught that only con men claim to be psychic or that only "gifted" people can use their intuition.

The truth is, we all are naturally intuitive. It is an integral part of our nature. With awareness and practice, it is possible to open up the energy of your third eye, your intuition. The courage to use your intuition arises from having the self-esteem to trust your instincts. To use your natural psychic ability you have to be able to ignore negative preconceived notions you have internalized and take your power back from other people's perceptions. This doesn't mean you should be gullible or naïve. Rather, you must have strong enough self-esteem to trust and act on the validity of what you are intuitively perceiving and override the censure of others. A positive self-image is essential for optimal use of your third eye.

When you are placed in a new situation or are meeting new people, tune into your energetic perception. How does it feel? What's your gut reaction? Asking yourself these kinds of questions and paying close attention to your energetic reactions to people and situations will hone your natural intuitive skill.

You are giving away your power in this energy center when you close your mind to new ideas or when you refuse to change your mind about beliefs that are damaging to you and those around you. Open-mindedness and tolerance are key. Even if you let new ideas into your consciousness, you are not obligated to adopt them. It is always your prerogative to reject concepts that don't empower you, but new ideas can stimulate growth and inspiration. It is damaging to close off the power of your mind completely by refusing to entertain concepts that might broaden your horizons. Ultimately, this refusal is fear-based. It causes you to block your intuition and relinquish your chi.

This is when attention and practice come in. Over time, you will notice which of your perceptions prove to be wrong and which ones are correct. One way you can separate a fear reaction from true intuition is by ascertaining the energetic "charge" that is associated with the thought. Does it feel loving or fearful? A truly intuitive perception will be infused with love rather than charged with fear. Since you are now adept at performing the Basic Power Practices and can differentiate between the energies of love and fear, you will be able to discern whether your intuition is valid.

If you are concerned that fear may cause you to misinterpret your intuitive messages, try using your intuitive sense first on the aspects of your life that don't involve momentous decisions. In this way, you can exercise and sharpen your intuition as you gain more confidence in your capacity to perceive its wisdom clearly.

Short Practice

If you feel your chi leaving your body from your forehead, pull the energy cord right back to you. When you feel that you want to use your intuition in a particular situation:

1. Straighten the spine and take a deep breath. Focus your awareness in the center of your forehead, picturing the color indigo.

2. Imagine your third eye opening up in the center of your forehead. Don't focus so much on the words that are being said in this particular situation. Instead, focus on the energy behind the words. What are you feeling? Keep your third eye open.

3. Allow yourself to trust your intuitive perceptions.

Level 1 Exercise

1. Sit on your heels on the floor. Lay your chest down on your knees, with your forehead and bridge of the nose on the floor. Your hands are lying at your sides, palms up.

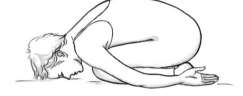

{ 1–2 }

2. Press your forehead to the floor. You are stimulating your intuition chakra. Let the spine stay loose and relax into this position, picturing the color indigo. Stay in this position for a while.

3. When you are ready, place your hands under your shoulders and push the upper body up. Focus on the energy flowing freely through your intuition chakra.

Just as you take the time physically to constrict and then release the pressure on the third eye to energize your Intuition Chakra, you can take a moment in your daily life to disengage mentally from a situation in order to listen to your inner wisdom.

Affirmation:
I let my mind relax so
that I can receive clear
messages from my intuitive
energy center.

Level 2 Exercise

1. Get on the floor on your hands and knees. Your spine should be parallel to the floor with your hands directly under the shoulders, knees under the hips.

2. Using the center of the forehead as your point of power, move the head downward so that you are looking at your thighs. Let the spine round up, following the movement of the head.

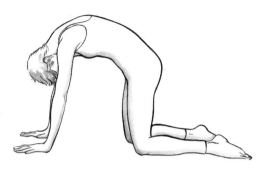

{ 1–2 }

3. Lift the forehead upward, looking at the ceiling, allowing the back to arch naturally.

4. Leading with your forehead, let it go in any direction you like, allowing the rest of the body to follow the movement of the head. You will feel as though you are giving yourself a back massage.

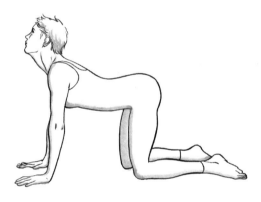

Just as the rest of the body falls into place as it follows the movement of your head, the rest of your life follows the lead of your intuition and falls joyfully into place.

{ 3 }

Affirmation:
I trust my intuition to
guide my decisions.

Level 3 Exercise

This practice should be done when you have already completed some other physical exercise so that the muscles are warm and ready to stretch. If your muscles are cold, replace this practice with Level 1 or Level 2.

1. Stand in a very wide stance, toes pointing forward, feet parallel. As you breathe in, lengthen the spine and straighten the arms out directly from your shoulders.

2. Exhale and lengthen your back as you hinge forward from the hips. Keeping the knees straight, lower the upper body all the way down, letting the hands hold on to the outsides of the ankles. If you can't lower your upper body enough to hold your ankles, hold on to the outsides of your legs as high up as necessary. Keep your back straight and look at the floor.

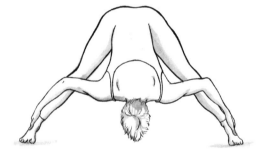

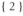

3. Lengthen the spine, leading with the center of the forehead toward the floor. Use the strength of your arms to pull on your legs to help lengthen the spine. You may or may not eventually get your forehead to the floor. It doesn't matter. Continue to reach toward the floor through the third eye. If your forehead is very far away from the floor, you can try placing your legs in a wider stance. If you can get your forehead to the floor, make sure that you are still pulling on your legs. *Do not put too much pressure on the head and neck.* If your forehead is on the floor, stay there for ten seconds.

4. To get out of this position, bend the knees while placing your hands on the floor directly under the

shoulders. Put all your weight on the hands. Walk the feet together. Soften the knees, push the feet into the floor, and roll up, slowly stacking the vertebrae one at a time as you straighten the spine.

Just as you lengthen your body in this exercise by leading with the center of your forehead (and eventually learn to balance your forehead on the floor), the perception of your third eye lights your path and can provide support and balance in your everyday life.

Affirmation:
I trust my intuition to support and lead me on
my right path.

To open your intuition energy center, you must trust in your innate intu-itiveness. Like anything else, it can be enhanced by awareness and practice.

Meditation and Practice: Opening the Third Eye

1. Get into a sitting position. Straighten the spine and breathe deeply. Take a moment to call your energy, your spirit, your thoughts into present time.

2. Focus your attention on your Intuition Chakra, located in the center of the forehead. Breathe into this energy center, visualizing the purplish blue color of indigo. As you continue to breathe into your intuition center, see the indigo color becoming more and more vibrant and radiant.

3. Using the index and middle fingers of the left hand, and visualizing a closed eye in the center of your forehead, gently press your fingers upward as though you were opening the eyelid of your third eye. Do this several times while continuing to breathe deeply, until you have a clear picture in your mind that your third eye is now open.

4. Send indigo light out of your third eye from your forehead and the back of the head. Send this light out from your intuition center with two clear intentions:
- To pick up subtle energy vibrations that you will be able to understand
- To open up your mind to higher concepts

5. With every breath you take, picture the indigo light of this energy center becoming clearer and brighter.

6. See your mind literally expand as it opens to accept higher wisdom.

7. Stay in this meditative state, feeling your sharpened intuition and under-standing. Trust that you have opened up your natural channel of heightened perception. When you feel ready, take another deep breath and open your eyes.

Chapter 18

THE UNITY CHAKRA

Color: Purple

Focus: Connection to the Divine

Point of Power: Top of the Head

The Unity Chakra represents our connection to a higher power and thus, to every other being. You may call your higher power *the Universe, Nature, God, or Divine Intelligence.* The name is immaterial. The idea is that there exists a point of power in the universe from which all beings, all planets, all solar systems originate. We are all *extensions* of this power source, whether we choose to acknowledge this connection or not. There are many ways to become more consciously aware of our connection with the divine: prayer, meditation, movement, the study of theology—the roads to travel are many, and all ultimately lead to the same place.

See what insights come to you when you focus on your Unity Chakra in meditation. You can also use your thoughts and intention to energize this chakra and intensify the vibrancy of its purple color. Don't hesitate to modify the spiritual philosophy of this chapter according to your own convictions. Explore what your own beliefs are regarding the nature of the universe. Perhaps you have an affinity for nature. You might do the meditations by using the idea that nature is the source for all living beings. Maybe you just want to focus on the fact that your family members all share a common ancestry, and use this to lead you to a sense of unity. The important thing to remember is that we do not exist in a vacuum. We are all connected to the divine and to every other being.

Short Practice

Any time you feel that you are relinquishing your chi from this energy center, pull the energy string back to you immediately. When you are in a situation in which you feel cast adrift and lost, take a moment to breathe deeply.

1. Draw your awareness to your Unity Chakra, picturing a radiant purple light. Imagine that you can open up the crown of your head and breathe in through your Unity Chakra. Transfer the sensation of breathing from your nose to the top of your head and see the light become more and more brilliant.

2. Say to yourself exactly how you feel in this moment, for example, "I feel lost," "I feel alone."

3. Send the purple light upward into the heavens with a request for help and comfort. Ask for exactly what you need: "I need comfort," "I need help."

4. Let that purple light shine down through your body. Be aware that you are heard, loved, and supported by the universe. You need only ask for assistance. Take another deep breath, and remember that you are *never* alone.

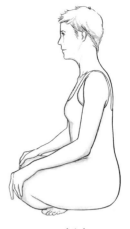

{ 1 }

Level 1 Exercise

1. Sit in a comfortable position, straightening the spine, relaxing, and breathing deeply.

2. Exhale, let the head drop forward, and allow the rest of the body to accommodate that movement. Your spine will naturally round out toward the back.

3. Inhale, then lift through the crown of the head as you straighten your back all the way through the tailbone.

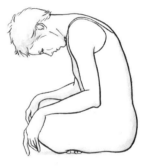

{ 2 }

Just as you allow the rest of your body to follow the motion of your head, in your life you "go with the flow" while listening for and receiving divine guidance.

Affirmation:
I go gracefully with what the
universe presents to me, trusting
that I am exactly where I'm
meant to be.

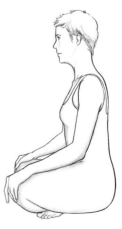

{ 3 }

Level 2 Exercise

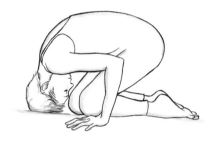

{ 1 }

1. Get on your knees on the floor and sit on your heels. Place your hands on the floor directly under the shoulders, round your back, and lower the crown of the head directly onto the floor. You will be looking at your stomach. Make sure you *do not put all of your weight* on your head. Most of your weight should be supported by your legs and hands, with only a gentle pressure at the top of the head.

In this exercise, you take a moment to put pressure on the crown of your head gently to block the energy flow. When you let go of that pressure by lifting your head, the energy rushes in with vigor and power. In order to hear your divine guidance clearly, you must take the time to become quiet and still. You can then receive direction with clarity and trust.

2. Visualize the color purple at the crown of your head. Allow your spine to stay rounded and relaxed. Feel a gentle stretch at the back of the neck. Stay with your full, relaxing breaths.

3. When you feel ready to stop the exercise, gently straighten your spine, pushing your hands into the floor as you raise your head and get back into the kneeling position.

Affirmation:
No matter what I'm doing, I can pause
for a moment to quiet my mind and
hear the voice of the Divine.

Level 3 Exercise

1. Start with your knees soft, feet hip distance apart. Leading with the top of the head, let it drop forward, allowing the knees to bend over the toes and the tailbone to slide backward.

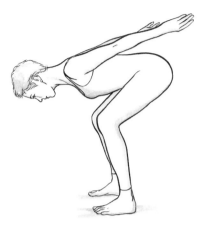

{ 1–2 }

2. Reach the arms down and back from the shoulders with your palms facing up. *Do not lower the body by using the back. Lower it by bending your legs.* You will end up looking as though you are going to dive into a swimming pool. Your thighs and tailbone are parallel to the floor, and your hands are reaching back. Reach through the crown of your head and through your tailbone to elongate your spine.

3. As you inhale, raise the head and lengthen the body up to a standing position. Lift the arms up over the head and rise up on the balls of the feet.

4. Repeat the exercise. As you exhale, drop the head and slide the tailbone back, reaching back with the arms.

5. Inhale by lengthening the body up in one motion, driving through the crown of the head. Continue with this practice until you feel that the Unity Chakra is more fully energized.

Just as you straighten the spine in one movement, reaching through the top of the head, you are aware that every muscle, every nerve in your body is connected. So it is in our lives. All beings are connected, and our actions effect everything and everyone around us.

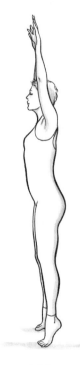

{ 3 }

Affirmation:
Everything I do and say ultimately affects those
around me. All beings are connected.

Meditation enables us to lose the sense of our physical boundaries and awaken to the reality that every being springs from the same energy source. We *are* divine energy. Our true nature is perfection. Although no human being is perfect, we are all manifestations of the same perfect energy. That is our authentic nature. Our bodies can be vulnerable to illness and our minds can be clouded by fear-based thoughts and emotions, but our spirit remains perfect no matter what our physical incarnation appears to be.

The more connected you are to your spiritual nature, the more you will act like the spiritual being you are. When you are disconnected from the truth of who you are, your actions will reflect that disconnection. Your spirit remains perfect no matter what you do and can always be a source of inspiration and guidance. It all depends on whether or not you listen and act in accordance with the energy of your soul.

Meditation and Practice
Oneness

1. Get into a sitting position and straighten your spine. Call your chi, your spirit, your thoughts into present time. Breathe deeply until you start to feel relaxed. Close your eyes. Focus your attention on the core of your body, seeing your light—brilliant, radiant, vibrant, and beautiful. Picture the purple hue at the crown of your head.

2. Visualize this light washing downward through every cell in your body, until your entire being radiates the same vibrant purple color. Acknowledge the perfection and beauty of your energy. Remember that you were

created perfect and perfect you remain. Nothing you could ever do or say could make you more perfect. Nothing you could ever do or say could make you less perfect. *Remember who you really are.*

3. As you recognize the divinity within you, acknowledge that every other being contains exactly the same light. Think of all the people you know. Look at them with the eyes of your spirit. See the same brilliant, perfect light in every one of them.

4. Go deep into yourself. Imagine that your consciousness is also going deep into the energy of everyone you know. As you go into your energy and the energy of all others, your consciousness journeys to the same source of brilliant, perfect, divine light from which all souls originate.

5. Stay in this light for as long as you like. When you are ready, take one more deep breath and open your eyes with an expanded awareness of the unity of all beings.

Your intuitive sense originates within you. Divine guidance is the direction that arises from whatever you conceive your higher power to be. Since we incarnate from the same divine source, intuition and divine guidance are really the same. However, the simple fact that we are in a physical incarnation gives us the perception that we are separate from our source. Therefore, we separate our guidance into individual (our spirit or soul) and universal (our source). Intuition comes from the knowledge of our soul, which in itself is divine. Divine guidance comes directly from the source of a higher power, which permeates our innermost being. The Unity Chakra is this connection's point of power. The clarity of our intuition and higher guidance reflects our connection with the divine.

Meditation and Practice
Divine Guidance

1. Lie on the floor with your spine straight. Close your eyes. Take deep, full, long breaths. Call your energy, your spirit, your thoughts into this moment. With every breath you take, feel your body let go of tension as you become more and more relaxed. Soon there is no holding anywhere in your body. You are totally relaxed.

2. Just as surely as your physical body is supported by the floor, your spirit is supported by the universe as you travel your path. Every person, every circumstance that enters your life is there to help you experience the lessons you need to learn, so that you can achieve your highest level of growth.

3. Dance with life and go gracefully with what the universe presents to you, knowing that you are exactly where you're meant to be, infinitely loved, supported, and guided every moment of your life.

"Going gracefully" means accepting with equanimity what you need to learn. It doesn't limit your conscious intention to achieve what you want. You create your reality both consciously and unconsciously, manifesting the lessons you need to learn in accordance with your spiritual growth.

Short Practice

As you go throughout your day, continue to hold the perception that every person who interacts with you is an enlightened teacher. Know that each person who touches your life offers you a lesson that is a gift.

(Keep in mind that not every gift seems desirable at first. Teachers often take unexpected forms. Look past outward appearances to the real meaning of each lesson.)

The following is an illustration of the miraculous in everyday life. We all have our wounds and our power losses. We must remember that in each moment, we are never alone. Forgiving ourselves is forgiving others. Healing ourselves helps to heal everyone.

Drew's Experience

The exercises and meditations for the Unity Chakra led Drew, my husband and partner, to an extraordinary revelation. As he sought to clarify his connection to the divine, one image appeared and persisted in his consciousness: a beatific human fetus, emanating light and love, compassion, and forgiveness. It evoked an intense reaction within Drew—at the same time electrifying and consoling his entire energy system. It looked like the celestial embryo at the climax of the film *2001,* and it communicated with Drew as if by telepathy, transmitting absolution and unconditional love. This didn't seem an act of his imagination. He could *feel* its presence and gradually became aware of its identity. It was Drew's brother. Not the younger brother he knew, but another sibling he had never been aware of, who infused Drew's soul with forgiveness and love and directed him to do the same for himself. Drew opened his eyes with astonishment, suddenly remembering what he had long forgotten—that his mother had suffered a miscarriage when he was three years old, two years before she gave birth to the boy Drew knew as his brother. Drew realized in an instant that much of the anxiety he had felt in his early development could be linked emotionally and energetically to this miscarriage. He confirmed with his mother that the miscarriage took place when he was three and that the unborn child had been a boy. Assimilating this revelation, he felt that he had purged his energy system, letting go of a primal fear that had blocked his growth, and clarified his connection to the divine unity of all experience. More than anything, Drew is filled with a daily sense of gratitude and appreciation, knowing that the passionate devotion and partnership he and I share, the joy of our creativity, and the miracle of our children all result from events set in motion for the evolution of our souls and signify the transcendence of love in the unity of all things.

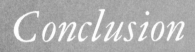

PART IV

Conclusion

The preceding chapters contain many tools to assist you on your journey to empowerment, healing, and spiritual growth. Remember to use whatever practices feel right for you. Don't judge your "performance." Treat yourself lovingly. These practices are meant to empower you. They are not another excuse to beat yourself up, so don't worry about doing them perfectly. Above all, as you draw the elements of Chi Fitness together to stay in your power and consciously create your reality, trust your instincts and allow your inner wisdom to show you the way.

Chapter 19

PUTTING IT ALL TOGETHER

As a child, I grew up in a home where we were not permitted to express negative feelings. My mother and father argued a lot, and I was terrified at a very early age that my parents would divorce. (They ultimately did.) I felt it was my job to make everybody happy in order to keep the peace. Therefore, I did everything I could to *appear* happy. Many times I wanted to cry, but I felt that if someone saw me cry, the shaky foundation of my family life would crumble. I literally learned to swallow my tears. It made my throat hurt, as though I were trying to swallow a rock. I didn't feel entitled or empowered enough to ask questions or express my panic.

I was giving away all of my power in the Voice Chakra by not speaking my truth. Therefore, I had very little chi in that area to keep it healthy. All my life, I have been prone to sore throats and strep infections. As an adult, I found it virtually impossible to express any feelings that were not positive. I always put a "good face" on whatever situation or relationship I found myself in, no matter how bad it was. No one except my best friend ever knew when I was unhappy, angry, or fearful.

As I became more aware of my energy system, I made the connection between my constant strep infections and my Voice Chakra. I began to force myself to say what I needed to say every chance I got. It was so hard for me. Every time I had to express my needs or my anger to someone I loved, I would go into a major panic. My heart would start to pound. I would be short of breath. I would physically have to "get a grip" by using the only power practice I knew at that time, taking deep, full breaths. Whenever I had to confront someone I had a relationship with, I was aware of my terror. It was the same terror that I felt when I was four years old. I was afraid that the person I was in relationship with would abandon me, just as I was afraid my parents would when I was four. The feeling was *exactly* the same except I was in a larger body.

When I made the connection between my extreme anxiety about confrontation as an adult and my childhood fears, I started using self-talk to take care of my four-year-old fears that never healed. I could also address my energy system by using the Power Practices for the Voice Chakra and using sounding in my meditation, as well as making an effort in my everyday life to give voice to my true emotions.

The important thing to remember is that *you and only you* are in charge of managing your chi. You can stay in your power or you can choose to give it away. There will always be times when you slip into fear. Now you know how to take your power back in a moment, then explore in more detail the roots of your fears. You can then start the process of healing yourself.

Elizabeth's Experience

Elizabeth is an artist who never considered herself to be a particularly spiritual person. She was drawn to Chi Fitness because she was looking for a different form of exercise, and she found that moving from the core of her body felt so much better than her usual workout. As Elizabeth's body started to open up, her emotions opened up, too, and her life began to change. In her new graphic arts business, she hired a young man who had a lot of ego. He was good at what he did, but he had an overblown sense of how talented he was. He would make outrageous demands and felt he was entitled to be a partner in Elizabeth's business, even though he had not yet made any significant contribution. As you might expect, he attracted clients who had very similar energy to his. And he lost a lot of them, too, as a result of his egotistical style. The clients who stayed were much like him, ego-driven and generally difficult to be around, attributes that Elizabeth now recognizes as fear-based. When Elizabeth refused to give in to him, he began to bad-mouth her behind her back, in her own office.

This was a new business for Elizabeth and she didn't want to fire him because he was bringing in some money. He was also a shameless womanizer and behaved inappropriately with female clients. Elizabeth tried to overlook it, rationalizing that these women were adults who knew what they were doing. She now sees that her decision *not* to fire him was totally fear-based. Elizabeth would become enraged with him and would have to keep pulling her power back at least ten times a day. Invariably, she felt the power loss most strongly in her Root Chakra, but she neglected to explore why. After a year of this nonsense, Elizabeth finally reached the end of her rope. She had wanted to fire him after the first three months. Now she knew she had to let him go, but she felt frozen. Why? Elizabeth sat with her feeling of fear and asked herself the Four Questions for Healing. She found that, in this situation, she felt she was twelve years old. When Elizabeth recalled her life when she was that age, she realized it was a period when her alcoholic father was bingeing nightly. All Elizabeth really wanted was for him to go away, but she was afraid for him to leave because her mother was ill-equipped to take care of Elizabeth and her six siblings. He was the breadwinner. His outrageous, nasty behavior was devastating to everyone in that house, but what would happen if he left? It was too scary to think about. And even as Elizabeth desperately wanted him to leave, she just as desperately needed him to stay. He was Dad and she longed for his positive presence in her life. The parallels between her employee and her father became obvious. Even though the loss of this young man really didn't mean a significant loss of income, he still reminded her of her father. That was why the fear was rising up.

Once Elizabeth realized the underlying dynamics of the situation, the difference in her reaction to this person was miraculous. She was able to ask him to leave in a civilized manner. There were some "blow-ups" and she would momentarily give her power to him, but since she was now aware of where her wounding was, Elizabeth could call her power back quickly and feel unruffled by these scenes. Instead of ruminating in anger over this person's behavior, she used self-talk and was now able to let it go and go on about her business. Elizabeth has continued to use these Power Practices, especially for the Root Chakra, and she feels much more grounded and secure in her business and her life.

There is yet another piece to this puzzle. By using the Power Practice, Spiritual Perspective, Elizabeth could see that this young man was offering her an important lesson. He was giving Elizabeth the opportunity to look at this very deep wound by activating it in her, so that she could begin to heal it. She can actually feel gratitude toward him because his behavior allowed her to grow in an important way. Elizabeth was also able to look at his behavior with compassion, knowing that whenever someone acts so unloving, his behavior is based in fear.

A Healing Journey through the Chakras

Here is another tool you can use when you have a moment to reflect on your fearful emotions. Take each fear-based thought and go through every one of your chakras. As you investigate your energy centers, picture the color of each one. Notice which colors are not bright and vibrant. This will indicate which chakras are affected by fear and need further work. If it is difficult to picture colors in your mind's eye, you may find it easier for you to sense whether the chi feels weak in any particular center. Again, this would indicate that more attention is needed in that chakra. These are useful tools for exploring imbalance of your energy system in every area of your life.

When you perceive how you feel about a conflict by identifying the sensations it produces in your body, you are in closer touch with your chi. This perception will enable you to be more precise about what is going on in your energy system and recognize which chakras could benefit most from further exploration.

Chakra Imbalances

Just as our energy affects other people, each chakra also affects every other chakra within our own energy systems. If you have an imbalance in one energy center, other centers will be off-balance as well. You can see this in the context of your own life. For instance, if you always felt emotionally overpowered as a child, your Root Chakra will undoubtedly have some energy blocks. This kind of stress in your early development would also cause you to relinquish your chi in the Internal Power Chakra, possibly resulting in poor self-esteem. It would follow that you could feel overpowered in your Voice Chakra and have trouble expressing yourself.

As another example, perhaps your childhood home was violent. This would cause you to relinquish energy in your Root Chakra. As an adult, you may exhibit violent behavior yourself, behavior that would indicate an imbalance in the External Power Chakra. You may also be giving away power in the Heart Chakra because you have learned that love hurts. An imbalance in the Voice Chakra would also result in a tendency to be verbally aggressive.

All of these imbalances can be corrected with awareness and practice, including professional therapy when necessary. As you heal one area of your energy system, the others will be affected as well. For example, if you have trouble speaking your truth, you can start to heal the Voice Chakra by using

Power Practices, asking the Four Questions for Healing, and simply saying what you need to say. This will help you feel better about yourself and automatically empower you to start regaining your energy in the Internal Power Chakra.

The important thing to remember is that when you reclaim your chi and correct any imbalance in one center of your energy system, you promote healing in the other centers as well.

In the following section we will explore each chakra in order to pinpoint specific problem areas in your energy system.

Root Chakra: Family of Origin Issues

Say you are having the experience of feeling rootless and disconnected from any kind of family system. This makes you frightened, so you clutch at any relationship you have, forcing the intimacy in order to feel grounded and have a sense of belonging. The people in your life start backing off because of the intensity of your neediness, which only reinforces your feeling of abandonment.

Lie down on a flat surface with your spine straight and close your eyes. Take deep, full, long breaths. Call your energy, your spirit, your thoughts into present time. Allow yourself to experience fully the depth of your emotion in relation to this issue.

Start at the *Root Chakra,* located between the tailbone and pubic bone, picturing the color red and sensing the vibrancy of your chi in this area.

- How does this bereft feeling compare with your feelings as a child?
- Were your parents physically present, but emotionally unavailable?
- How does this emotional conflict regarding family bonds compare to what you lived through as a child?

Now, attend to your *External Power Chakra* between the pubic bone and the belly button. Visualize the color orange and feel your chi in this chakra.

- As a child were you permitted to express your creativity?
- Were you able to feel as though you had power or significance in your family?
- What kind of a bond, if any, did you have with anyone in your family? Were you always in a subservient position?

Focus your attention on the *Internal Power Chakra.* In your mind's eye, see the color yellow in the solar plexus. Feel the energy in this center.

- How did your family of origin effect your self-esteem?
- Can you praise and see value in yourself without looking to others to define you?
- Do you have an internal value system developed by you, or did you fully adopt the values of your tribe?

Travel now to the *Heart Chakra* at the center of your chest, picturing the color green. Notice how your chi feels in this area.

- As you were growing up, was love given freely or was it conditional?
- Was there any kind of abuse, subtle or not, that taught you to close your heart as a way of avoiding pain?
- Was it difficult to feel compassion for anyone in your family because of your own victimization?

Draw your attention up to the *Voice Chakra* at the base of your throat, seeing the color blue in your mind's eye, and perceive the energy in this center.

- When you were growing up, were you permitted to speak your truth?
- Were you allowed a certain amount of autonomy?

- Could you authentically express the full range of your emotions, whether they were positive or not?

Focus on the *Intuition Chakra* at the center of your forehead. Visualize the color indigo (bluish purple), sensing the chi in this chakra.

- Now that you are older, can you use the reasoning of your intellect to understand why you are having this particular conflict at this time in your life?
- Can you look deeper, using your third eye, to see the true motivation for your family's behavior?

Finally, move up to the *Unity Chakra* at the crown of your head. Picture the color purple and sense your chi in this center.

- In the midst of your pain concerning your feeling of not belonging, can you understand that whatever happened in your family, your spirit selected them precisely for the lessons you are now having to face?
- Can you accept that these souls with whom you grew up are a part of you and contain exactly the same perfect light as you?

As you finish progressing through your chakra system, take note of any centers that seemed dull in color or less vital than the others. You will want to look deeper into the issues governed by these energy centers. You can ask yourself the *Four Questions for Healing* to delve further into the issues that you find during this journey through the chakras. The following is a modified version of the Four Questions that fits more specifically into this practice:

1. As I traveled through the chakras, when I came upon an issue to which I had relinquished my chi, how old did I feel?
2. What happened when I was that age?

3. How is that past situation similar to the current one I am now exploring?

4. How will I take my power back?

The fourth question here offers a choice about which Power Practices you will use to heal yourself. You can use *Power in Present Time, Reclaiming Your Chi,* the appropriate *Chakra Power Practices,* and *Spiritual Perspective.* In other words, use any practice or exercise that feels right to you.

Chi Fitness can be physically and emotionally challenging. Feeling "stretched" in your body or your psyche can be stimulating—but it can also be intimidating, even threatening. These practices should always feel safe and encourage your growth. Don't feel you have to do them alone. Feelings are bound to come to the surface as you free up your chi, and managing them properly may include the support of friends and family or a professional therapist.

The following is an exercise that you can take your time with or use as a Short Practice to energize your chakra system by using conscious movement and visualization.

Conscious Movement Chakra Meditation and Practice

1. Get into a sitting position with your spine straight and eyes closed. Take deep, full, long breaths. Call your energy, your spirit, your thoughts back from everything that is not here and now. Feel the sensation of being fully in your power and present in this moment.

2. Move your attention to the Root Chakra. Breathe through this chakra at the perineum. Using the perineum as your point of power, move it any way you want, allowing the rest of your body to follow this motion. (This movement can be subtle or vigorous.) As you work with the Root Chakra, visualize the chi as becoming more energetic, and the color red more intense.

3. Move up to the lower abdomen and the External Power Chakra. Imagine that there is a balloon in your lower body. Breathe through this area as if you were blowing up and expanding the balloon with every inhalation. When you exhale, feel it deflate and contract. As you continue with this movement, see in your mind's eye the color orange becoming brighter and more vibrant.

4. Go up to your solar plexus and your Internal Power Chakra. Using your rib cage as your point of power, push it forward as you breathe in, and backward as you breathe out. Then move it any way you like, remembering to breathe deeply and easily. Picture the color yellow becoming more brilliant and energized.

5. Move your awareness up to the Heart Chakra in the center of your chest. As you breathe in, open the chest outward as though there were a hinge in the center of your body. As you exhale, open up the space between your shoulder blades. In your mind's eye, see the color green getting more vibrant and radiant.

6. Move your attention up to the Voice Chakra at the base of your throat. Breathe in, contracting the back of your neck so that your head drops backward. Then contract the front of your neck so that your chin drops down toward the chest as you exhale. Picture the color blue becoming more vibrant and intense.

7. Go upward to the Intuition Chakra in the center of your forehead. As you breathe through this center, use the index and middle fingers of your left hand to push up on your forehead gently as though you were opening the eyelid of your third eye. Visualize the indigo color becoming more radiant and brilliant.

8. Finally, raise your awareness to the crown of your head and the Unity Chakra. Breathe through this energy center. Move the top of your head in

any direction, allowing the rest of your body to follow. See in your mind's eye the color purple, bright and energetic. Let that purple color shine down through every cell of your body, so that you are bathed in beautiful purple light.

9. Use all of the seven chakras in the core of your body, from the tailbone to the crown of your head, as one vertical point of power. As you breathe in, arch your back, raising your chin and letting your head drop backward. As you exhale, round your back and let your head drop forward. Feel your body opening and closing from its core with every breath you take. Be aware of the perfect balance of your energy system. Resolve to go through your day remembering who you really are and recognizing the perfection of all others as well.

External Power Chakra
Power Struggles

Here we will work with the scenario that you are having major power struggles with your preadolescent or adolescent child. (Keep in mind that you can use this practice with any relationship by modifying the questions.)

Lie down on a flat surface with your spine straight and close your eyes. Take deep, full, long breaths. Call your energy, your spirit, your thoughts into present time. Think of the essence of your power struggle with your child. Think of a specific incident or sequence of events that troubles you and get a sense of what the power struggle feels like in your body.

Focus your awareness on your *Root Chakra.* Picture the color red and sense the vibrancy of the chi in this chakra.

- Ask yourself what this conflict has to do with *your* family of origin. How is it familiar?
- Did you as a child feel the same way you do now?
- Can you identify with the way your child is feeling?

Draw your attention to your *External Power Chakra.* See in your mind's eye the color orange and sense your chi in this area.

- How does this conflict with your child make you feel about your power over him?
- Are you afraid for his safety, or are you fearful of allowing him to make decisions because that threatens your authority? Be honest with yourself.

Move your consciousness to your *Internal Power Chakra,* picturing the color yellow. Sense your energy in this center.

- Does this problem with your child have to do with your sense of self?
- Do you have a lot invested in his behavior?
- Do you want him to act the way you did at that age?
- Does his acting out embarrass you?
- Do you feel that his behavior is a reflection on you that others will judge?

Go now to the *Heart Chakra.* Visualize the color green and sense the chi in this center.

- Is your conflict with your child allowing you to feel love and compassion for the life changes he is experiencing?
- Are you judging his behavior as wrong without being able to feel empathy?
- Are you loving him enough to be able to put up a loving boundary around his behavior toward you?
- Are you compassionate toward yourself when you react to him?

Now up to the *Voice Chakra,* visualizing the color blue. Discern whether the chi in this chakra is weak or vibrant.

- Are you speaking your truth to your child without trying to manipulate him?
- Are you trying to impose your will on him?
- Is his behavior controlling you?
- Are you able to communicate with him in a loving manner that is from your heart and balanced with the intelligence of your mind?

Move your awareness up to the *Intuition Chakra.* Picture the color indigo and feel the chi in this energy center.

- In this situation with your child, are you using not only your intellect, but your intuition as well?
- Are you looking deeper than what is apparent on the surface?
- Are you able to look past what may seem like bravado and discern any confusion or fear that your child is really feeling?

Finally, move your attention to your *Unity Chakra.* Picture the color purple. Sense the chi in this chakra.

- Are you actively seeking divine guidance?
- At the most difficult moments with your child, are you acknowledging that this is all part of the journey the two of you are meant to take together?
- Are you mindful that you are, in addition to being his caretaker and nurturer, also your child's spiritual custodian, modeling lessons that will be with him forever?
- Are you aware of the connection between the two of you, remembering that you both carry the identical light?

Take note of the chakras that seemed to be most affected by the power struggle with your child and look deeper into any issues that should be examined. Any healing you do within yourself will also be healing for your child and your relationship. This process allows you to take back your power from any fear-based thinking that surrounds the conflict, freeing up the energy for both of you to grow and learn from it.

Internal Power Chakra: Self-Esteem Issues

Are you always walking around berating yourself? Do you feel inferior? Are you afraid to do what you really want because you don't think you deserve to be happy? Do you feel incapable of succeeding? When someone mildly criticizes you, do you feel you've been punched in the solar plexus? These are all indications that you are accustomed to relinquishing your power.

Lie down on a flat surface with your spine straight and close your eyes. Take deep, full, long breaths. Call your energy, your spirit, your thoughts into this moment. Explore your true feelings about yourself and your capabilities. Get a sense of how this feels in your body.

Focus your consciousness on your *Root Chakra.* See the color red and notice how your chi feels in that area.

- How were you made to feel in your family of origin?
- Were you important to the family system, or did you feel insignificant?
- Were you encouraged to follow your own path?
- Were your parents always expressing too much concern about you, so that you ended up feeling unable to take care of yourself?
- Was the underlying message in your family that you really weren't bright or talented?

Direct your awareness to the *External Power Chakra,* sensing the color orange and your chi in this chakra.

- As a child, were you able to strike out on your own without interference?
- Were you surrounded by teachers in school who were supportive or overbearing?

- Were your peers extremely critical of you?
- When you were a teenager, could you accept the bodily changes occurring within you, or were you relentlessly hard on yourself?

Go now to your *Internal Power Chakra.* Visualize the color yellow, feeling the chi in this chakra.

- Do you live your life by your own beliefs or do you usually follow the directions of others?
- Are you living your life in alignment with your deepest desires?

Move on to the *Heart Chakra.* Perceive the color green and the chi in this chakra.

- Are you able to be compassionate with yourself?
- Can you accept that you make mistakes, or do you chastise yourself unmercifully?
- Do you feel worthy to receive love from someone who is your equal?
- Can you accept and understand that you are a blessing to everyone your life touches?
- Do you believe that your love and compassion can heal others?

Travel up to the *Voice Chakra,* picturing the color blue, sensing the chi at the base of your throat.

- When you speak about yourself, do you use a self-deprecating tone?
- Do you subtly insult yourself?
- Can you speak your truth while honoring, yet not surrendering to, the beliefs of others?

Move your attention now to the *Intuition Chakra.* Visualize the color indigo, and sense your chi here.

- Can you use the power of your mind to take a good look at your worth, acknowledging your assets honestly and without shame?
- Can you use your intuition to remember who you are, to connect with the perfection of your spirit?

Go now to the *Unity Chakra,* picturing the color purple and sensing the chi in that energy center.

- Do you remember having the experience of feeling disconnected from any source?
- Have you felt that true union with another was only for special people, not you?
- Can you remember that everyone carries the same magnificent, divine light and that yours is just as perfect and brilliant as all the others?

Once again, attend to the chakras that seemed most affected by poor self-esteem and ask the Four Questions for Healing. Use whatever Power Practices empower you most.

Heart Chakra
Opening the Heart

In this example, you want to open your heart to an individual with whom you'd like to have an intimate relationship. You are trying very hard to do this, but you just can't seem to stay open and loving. Every time you start to feel love for him, you automatically do something that will alienate him. You want to understand this behavior. Once again, start by lying down on a flat surface with your spine straight. Close your eyes and take deep, full, long breaths. Call your energy, your spirit, your thoughts into present time. Allow yourself to reexperience all of the times when you have closed off your heart to love. In your body, get the general feeling of the fear that accompanies your shutting down.

Starting with the *Root Chakra,* sense the color red and feel the chi within that energy center.

- What was love like in your family home as you grew up?
- Was it demonstrative and open, or was it aloof and withdrawn?
- Was it overwhelming and smothering?
- Was there some type of abusive behavior going on, so that you learned to associate love with pain?

Draw your consciousness to your *External Power Chakra,* picturing the color orange and perceiving the chi in this area.

- Were there times in your life when you tried to demonstrate your love to someone, only to experience trauma?
- Were you manipulated by someone because you loved her?
- Do you equate loving someone with losing yourself?

Now go up to your *Internal Power Chakra,* visualizing the color yellow. Sense the chi in this chakra. Look deeply into your opinion of yourself.

- Do you feel that you are not worthy of having a relationship?
- Or are you afraid that if you open your heart, you will find that it is incapable of experiencing love?

Move your attention to your *Heart Chakra,* picturing its green color and feeling the chi in this center.

- Do you feel that if you open your heart, someone is bound to break it?
- Are you afraid that loving somebody will make you vulnerable and weak?
- Did you learn somehow that love equals pain?
- Can you have compassion for yourself in this conflict?

Direct your awareness to your *Voice Chakra,* visualizing the color blue and perceiving the chi in this energy center.

- Can you tell a dear one how you feel about him?
- Do affectionate words come easily or do they stick in your throat?
- When you think about saying something loving to someone, do you automatically start to feel afraid?
- In the past, did you verbalize your love to someone, only to have it culminate in a painful experience?

Now progress to your *Intuition Chakra,* picturing the color indigo and feeling the chi in this chakra. Try using your third eye. Look beyond appearances to see the gift or lesson you need to embrace in order to have a loving relationship in your life now.

- Can you use your intellect to look at your life up to now and understand why you have a hard time opening your heart?
- Can you see what has blocked your ability to love?
- Can you understand your fear?

Last, move your attention up to the *Unity Chakra.* In your mind's eye, see the color purple and sense the chi in that center.

- Can you see that the light and perfection that infuse you are also in every other person?
- Can you see that everyone has fear around certain loving relationships, that there is always the chance of getting hurt?
- Can you see that every single person in your life is worth loving?
- Can you accept this truth and unplug from your fear-based emotions?

Look closer at the chakras that are most affected by your fear of letting love into your life. Use the Four Questions, reclaim your chi, and energize these chakras with the Power Practices.

Voice Chakra
Issues of the Voice and Will

Perhaps you have a difficult time verbalizing your true emotions. Maybe you shrink from any kind of a debate because you are afraid that you'll say something stupid. Do you hesitate to disagree with the opinions of your friends? Do you feel anxious if you ask for what you need in a relationship? When you are upset with your loved one, do you hold back your feelings? Do you have a hard time telling anyone what you want? Does it frighten you to use your will in a way that others don't agree with? If any of these descriptions sounds like you, then you have work to do in this energy center. Lie down on a flat surface with your spine straight. Close your eyes and take deep, full, long breaths. Call your energy, your spirit, your thoughts into present time. Take a moment to feel the fear that accompanies the act of speaking your truth or exercising your will.

Draw your consciousness to the *Root Chakra,* sensing the red color and the energy in this chakra.

- In your family of origin, were you allowed to exert your will, or were you overly controlled by your caregivers?
- Were you allowed to express anger and sadness, or did you feel that you always had to pretend to be happy?
- Was there a lot of yelling and conflict in your household?

Bring your attention now to the *External Power Chakra,* visualizing the color orange and perceiving the chi in that area.

- Have you been around others who imposed their will on you?
- Did you resist their domination?
- If so, was their love for you conditional on whether you acquiesced?
- Did you ever use your voice to let your will be known, only to end up hurt and humiliated?
- Have you ever tried to dominate someone else?

Travel up to the *Internal Power Chakra*, picturing the color yellow and sensing the energy in that chakra.

- Have you ever summoned the courage to speak in a crowd and said the wrong thing?
- Did it upset you so much that you could think of little else for days afterward?
- Have you ever been unable to verbalize your original ideas?
- Are you unable to express the need to be nurtured?

Go now to your *Heart Chakra*, sensing its green color and the chi in this chakra.

- Can you speak your truth from your heart?
- Can you verbalize your positive and negative emotions?

Move your awareness now to the *Voice Chakra*, visualizing the color blue and feeling your chi in this center.

- Have you ever completely given your will over to someone or something outside yourself?
- Have you ever tried to control someone else totally through manipulative words?
- Are you addicted to a substance or obsessed with someone?

Go upward now to the *Intuition Chakra*, picturing the color indigo and perceiving the energy in this chakra. With the reasoning of your intellect, look back on your life and see whether you can realize why you have a difficult time using your voice and exerting your will.

- Has your mind censored your voice, taking its cue from your fear?
- What can you learn from all the times you have not spoken but felt that you should have? Use the power of your intuition to try to comprehend why this lesson has been given to you.

Direct your attention now to the *Unity Chakra,* seeing in your mind's eye its purple color and sensing the chi of this energy center.

- Have you ever been unable to express your feeling of unity with another?
- Have you ever tried to verbalize your belief in the unity of all people or your belief in a higher power and felt that you would be ridiculed?

See whether you can work on the chakras that are most dramatically affected by voice and will issues. Energize all your chakras, remembering to be kind to yourself. In order to heal your wounds you must treat yourself with kindness, not criticism.

Intuition Chakra
Issues That Block Intuitive Guidance

If you're like most people, it's difficult for you to trust your intuition. Even when you intuit something accurately, you're likely to discount it. If you do, you are depriving yourself of an extraordinary channel of information. To cultivate your intuition, all you need to use are awareness and practice. Like a muscle that hasn't been exercised, intuition atrophies with nonuse. Once you begin to apply your intuitive sense, it will become second nature to you. Lie down on a flat surface with your spine straight. Close your eyes and take deep, full, long breaths. Call your energy, your spirit, your thoughts into this moment. Gather all the sentiments you've had about your intuition—the times you have been right, the times when you've denigrated it. Get a feeling in your body about your intuitive sense.

Start with the *Root Chakra,* sensing the color red and the chi in this center.

- In your family of origin was every issue either black or white, with no middle ground?
- Did your family believe in only what they could see, feel, hear, smell, and taste?

- Was there any room for magical thinking in your household?
- Was your family rooted in religious doctrine that prohibited other points of view?

Direct your consciousness to the *External Power Chakra,* seeing in your mind's eye the color orange and feeling the chi in this center.

- Were you surrounded by authority figures who ridiculed anything that couldn't be perceived by the five senses?
- Were you taught by rote rather than by your own exploration?
- Were you allowed to question dogma, or was independent thinking frowned upon?

Go up to the *Internal Power Chakra,* visualizing the color yellow and perceiving the chi in this chakra.

- Do you have strong enough self-esteem to trust your gut feelings?
- Can you honor your intuition and follow it against the advice of those around you?

Now travel to the *Heart Chakra,* sensing the color green and the energy in this center.

- Can you allow your intuition to instruct you to follow your heart without fear?
- Does your intuitive sense inspire you to have compassion for others despite their surface behavior?
- Have you ever ignored your intuition about someone's love for you?

Direct your attention now to your *Voice Chakra.* Picture the blue color of this center and sense the chi in it.

- Can you assert your will enough to act out what your intuition has told you?
- Are you able to verbalize that your reasons for acting as you do are guided by your intuitive feelings?

Move upward to your *Intuition Chakra,* seeing the color indigo in your mind's eye and perceiving the chi in this center.

- Have you had an intuitive insight and used logic to talk yourself out of it?
- If something miraculous happens, do you deny it by trying to explain it away?

Go now to the *Unity Chakra,* visualizing the color purple, sensing the chi in this chakra.

- Can you comprehend that intuitive guidance and divine guidance both originate in the same source?
- Do you feel that your intuition is from your soul, which is connected to the universal consciousness of all sentient beings?

Remember which chakras are most affected by your doubts about your intuition. Do the practices for those chakras and the other Power Practices that feel right to you.

Unity Chakra
Separation

Have you always had the feeling that you are spiritually alone on this Earth? Are you convinced that when your body dies, every aspect of your existence dies with it? Do you feel disconnected from most people? Do you reject the idea of a higher power or creative source? If you would like to explore the avenue governed by this energy center, start by lying down on a flat surface with your spine straight. Close your eyes and take deep, full, long breaths. Call your energy, your spirit, your thoughts into present time. Feel all the emotions that arise up concerning your connection to the divine.

Sense in your body these thoughts and feelings, and draw your awareness to your *Root Chakra,* perceiving the color red and the energy there.

- As you were growing up, did your family have strong religious beliefs?
- If so, did you accept or reject them?
- Were they a help or a hindrance?
- Was your family tolerant of other faiths?

Go now to the *External Power Chakra.* Picture the color orange and feel the energy in this chakra.

- Did people around you say your thoughts and urges were sinful?
- Is it your sense that religions control believers through guilt and fear?
- Do you feel entitled to question religious and spiritual concepts?

Move your consciousness to the *Internal Power Chakra,* seeing the yellow color in your mind's eye and feeling the energy in this chakra.

- Did you internalize the judgments of others, believing your true nature to be inherently sinful?
- Are you unable to trust in a higher power because of the suffering in the world?
- Does this lead you to trust only yourself?

Move upward to the *Heart Chakra,* visualizing the color green and sensing the chi in this chakra.

- Can you forgive yourself for making mistakes and transfer that kindness to others, realizing that at our core we are all the same?
- Do you feel that you must protect yourself by closing your heart?

Direct your attention to the *Voice Chakra,* seeing the color blue in your mind's eye and perceiving your energy in this center.

- Have you ever been punished for questioning the existence of a higher force in our lives?
- Are you hesitant to give voice to your core beliefs?

Travel to the *Intuition Chakra,* visualizing the color indigo while sensing the energy in this chakra.

- Has your intuitive sense led you to feel a connection with someone?
- Did you honor the feeling or push it aside?
- Have you ever understood what another person was feeling without a word being said, even if you just met?

Finally, go to the *Unity Chakra,* picturing the color purple and feeling the chi at the crown of your head.

- Have you ever felt a sense of oneness with someone, only to be devastated when the relationship fell apart?
- Do you think you may have received divine guidance but chose to invalidate it because of fear?
- When you contemplate the universe, do you feel connected or disconnected?
- Do you gravitate toward a sense of isolation or unity with all things?

As always, recognize which of your energy centers are most influenced by this conflict. Select the Power Practices that you have an affinity for, reclaim your chi, and let go of your fear.

Reenergizing the Chakras

Once you are finished working your way through your chakra system, take the time to energize each energy center with the intention of reclaiming your chi:

1. Direct your awareness to your Root Chakra, at the perineum. Allow your awareness to wash over this energy center. Have the intention of using this washing action as you would an ocean wave, clearing away blocks and invigorating the red color of this chakra by making it brighter and more vibrant. Progress upward through the rest of the chakras:

2. External Power Chakra in the lower abdomen, working with the color orange.

3. Internal Power Chakra and the color yellow.

4. Heart Chakra and the color green.

5. Voice Chakra and its blue color.

6. Intuition Chakra with the color indigo.

7. Unity Chakra and the color purple.

This exercise will reenergize your energy system, leaving you feeling vibrant and peaceful.

Chapter 20

STAYING IN YOUR POWER

Experiencing the unity of your chi, body, and mind allows you to know the truth of who you are. This conscious awareness keeps you in your power and in the moment.

Many people live their lives unconscious of the wisdom of the body and the power of chi. As we have been discussing throughout this book, the mind, body, and chi are one; they cannot be separated. We only think they are separate when we live primarily in our intellect, insensible to what our bodies and energy systems are telling us.

Chi Fitness is about honoring the unity of your body, mind, and life force energy and managing this network on a daily basis to improve every aspect of your life. You can use this knowledge to heal old wounds, to improve the quality and depth of your relationships, and to help you live your life in ways that are based in love and not fear.

As you use conscious movement, you increasingly trust the innate intelligence of the body. You become more aware of your chi, recognizing where in your body it is blocked and where it is free-flowing. Your intellect then processes the information from your body and energy system and relates it to the larger context of your life. As you practice consciously moving your body and your chi, you make these Power Practices your own.

It doesn't matter what your body looks like while you are doing these physical exercises; it only matters how you *feel*. As you unblock and direct the flow of chi in your body through movement, thought, and meditation, your life flows naturally into a better place. You become aware of the unity of your body, chi, mind and spirit, and that awareness leads the way to deeper self-knowledge and healing. Controlling your weight, getting in better shape, and curtailing stress also result when you empower yourself with these practices.

There are many factors that contribute to our dissatisfaction with our appearance. We often empower food more than we empower ourselves. We may have self-esteem problems, or we may use food as a substitute for comfort. When you use these Power Practices and start to manage your energy, you will uncover and understand your own behavior better. You will open up your energy system, and that may lessen your food cravings and tendency to overeat. You will be more likely to know when you need to stop eating because you will be more sensitive to when you are full.

Whatever form of movement you enjoy, when you direct your focused attention to the activity your body is performing, you will discover new ways to improve your own style. This process is not about judging yourself. No matter what shape you're in, whether you are an expert or a beginner, conscious awareness will vastly improve your facility in any activity.

There is a difference between being aware of what's going on in your body and *judging* it, making yourself wrong. Don't worry about how "good" or "bad" you look or compare your performance to that of others. Your body will always communicate what activity level feels right. Stay at whatever level works for you. Using conscious movement, you will learn how to challenge yourself without risking injury. If you go to your fitness class after not getting enough sleep, listen to that fatigue, even if you're a seasoned athlete. It's your body sending a message to you. Stay at Level 1. On the other hand, if you are feeling extremely energetic, then progress to Level 3. In group exercise, people can get discouraged because they compare their performance to that of others and end up judging themselves harshly. If you are tired and choose to remain at Level One, you are not only doing yourself a great service; you are also helping others around you. If another person is feeling fatigued and he notices you honoring yourself by exercising at the beginning level, you give that person permission to do the same. You actually make it a "safe place" for that person to be in. In the same vein, if you are reluctant to go full speed because you're afraid that others will think you are showing off, realize that by allowing yourself to excel, you give others permission to shine, too. In both scenarios, you are an inspiration to the people around you.

Joy arises when you can acknowledge the truth of who you are. When you move your power into present time, you can be loving and accepting of yourself. You are in your power and filled with contentment. You aren't troubled about the past or worried about the future. You are not making negative judgments about yourself. You are fully present, in your power, and connected to your natural state of being, which is joy.

But what if you're in a state of pain or anguish—right now?

It's always essential to acknowledge your feelings, both physical and emotional, fully. Acknowledging the truth of what you are experiencing is, in itself, an act of love and self-acceptance and is especially important in times of anguish. It is possible to alleviate physical pain by managing your chi, but this usually takes many years to master. There is nothing wrong with seeking appropriate medical attention for physical or emotional pain. In the words of Dr. Andrew Weil, who says in *Sound Body, Sound Mind,* "The body wants to be healthy and is always trying to restore balance when balance is lost, but the circumstances of illness or injury can overwhelm its capacity to do so. In such cases, outside help—treatment—can be welcome, even lifesaving. It is important to understand the distinction between treatment and healing: treatment comes from outside, while healing comes from within."

These Power Practices can help you achieve a natural state of health and inner peace, but this is a process of learning, not a spontaneous burst of enlightenment. Always remember how important it is not to judge yourself or your progress in this regard. Treat yourself with the nurturing respect you deserve. When you can be compassionate toward yourself, you are an inspiration to be around, since you are then able to extend that loving acceptance to others. It is your natural state of being.

Meditation and Practice
Joy

1. Sit or lie with your spine straight in a comfortable position. Close your eyes. Call your chi, your spirit, your thoughts into the present moment. Breathe in brilliant, radiant, clear, healing light. Let that light circulate deeper and deeper into your body with every breath you take.

2. When you feel peaceful and present, let your consciousness go deep into the core of your body. At the core of your being are love, light, and joy. Find that place of joy and power that is central to your being, and enjoy feeling the peaceful happiness in this relaxed place.

3. Memorize how the pulsation of joy feels. Allow that feeling to expand outward through your body and past the physical limits of your body. Be aware of the vibration of joy, power, and light through your physique.

4. You now embody joy. You have drawn the happiness that is your true nature into your physical being. This is who you are.

Open your eyes and go forward into your day, embodying your true nature.

Short Practice

Take a deep breath, sending your awareness deep inside your body. Find the joy and light that are you. Expand them outward so that you can embody your true self. Whatever you do now, whether it is exercise or a business meeting, originates in the truth of your joyful spirit.

When you learn how to manage your energy, it follows naturally that your life will improve. Being in your power means making choices every moment of your life from the intention of love rather than fear. Ultimately, it is because of fear that we relinquish our power. Being empowered does not mean being selfish or self-absorbed. It doesn't mean usurping the power of other people. When you are truly in your power, you automatically honor the self-empowerment of others as well.

When we are jealous and try to denigrate another person's achievements, we are giving away our chi by being afraid that her success will detract from our own. In that moment, we need to realize that our potential is infinite and there is room for everyone's success. Remembering this helps us to stay in our power.

Love, too, is limitless. Only fear is limiting. When you open your heart to the infinite nature of love, you will find that jealousy and envy no longer have any power over you. The following passage paraphrases a beautiful exercise by Jane Nelsen in the audiotape *Building Self-Esteem Through Positive Discipline*, intended to be used when your older child is feeling insecure about a new baby. It applies, as well, to any kind of adult relationship.

The Infinite Nature of Love

Take out three candles, one candle to symbolize you (the parent), one for your older child, and one for your younger child. Light the candle that represents you and say, "See this flame? This flame is all my love. When you were born, I gave you all my love." (Using your candle, light the candle that represents your older child.) "And see, you've got all my love, but I still have all my love left. Now when the baby was born, I gave her all my love, too." (Light the baby's candle with the flame from your candle.) "But see, I still have all my love, you have all my love, and the baby has all my love, too. Love multiplies. Every time you give it away, you have more to give."

When you allow yourself to be who you really are, you are a gift to all those who enter your life. When you speak your truth, it is a blessing and an inspiration to everyone around you, giving him or her permission to do the same. We stay in our power when we can allow our children to have their own opinions and make their own mistakes. We empower ourselves when we hold the space for our partners to follow their hearts and explore their true nature. In fact, *when we empower ourselves, we empower everyone around us.*

When we follow our hearts, we empower ourselves. We realize that our talents are distinctive and are meant to be shared with the world. We are empowered when we find joy in what we do for a living and provide services from the heart that are uniquely our own.

All work is service to others and to yourself. When you feel anxious about your job performance, try to remember that underrating your talents is just as bad as being arrogant about them. *Your work is not about you alone.* Every person whose life you touch through your career will, in turn, take that positive energy and pass it on in some way to others. Every loving thought and kind gesture you incorporate into your life's work will influence more people than you could ever imagine.

A Personal Note

There have been times when I've stood in front of a really large Chi Dance class not knowing most of the people in the room. I start to get nervous about whether I'll be good enough to give them what they need and want. What I have to remember at those times is that these people were led to me for a reason. My task is simply to present what I know. It's not about me. It's not about how talented or untalented I am. It's about whatever these people came for that they will take with them when they leave. This keeps me out of my ego and fear and in a space of service and love.

Meditation and Practice
Staying in Your Power

1. Sit or lie in a comfortable position with your spine straight. Take deep, full breaths. Close your eyes and call your energy, your spirit, your thoughts into present time. Breathe in radiant, clear, brilliant, healing light. Visualize that it is rushing, streaming into every cell, every nerve, every muscle fiber. With every breath you take, you are becoming more radiant, clear, and relaxed.

2. Take a moment to remember who you really are. Feel your chi running through your entire body. Notice the feeling of peaceful calm that empowers you in this moment. Acknowledge the brilliance of your light.

3. Staying in your power means that you are fully present in the moment and are not afraid. You are aware that you manage and direct your energy. You can send it out with a loving intention or give it away through fear.

4. You can choose to take back your power at any time. You are completely in charge of where you place your chi.

5. You are a perfect, magnificent being and you recognize this in everyone else. You can project the truth of your power and dazzling light out into the world.

6. See in your mind's eye the brilliant, vibrant light at the core of your body. Recognize this light as your essence of pure joy. Use your intention to expand that light outward past the physical limits of your body. You are now surrounded by beautiful light.

7. Expand your light even farther to encompass the entire room. Enlarge your light to the size of the building. Send your light outward with the intention of love, so that everyone that comes into contact with it benefits from your loving energy.

8. Reach your light out farther to encompass your entire city. Keep making your light bigger to envelop more and more space.

9. Realize that the power of your energy doesn't diminish as you continue to send it out with loving intent. Continue to expand outward to encompass your country and then the world. Feel your expansive energy and the power of your light.

10. Stay in this space for as long as you like. When you are ready, draw your energy and light back to your physical body, affirming that energy is not bound by time or space.

11. Take a few more moments to *feel* the truth of how powerful, how significant you are. Remember and acknowledge that you are a precious gift to every person your life touches. Stay centered in the truth of who you are.

Give yourself a moment and then open your eyes. You are radiant, powerful, peaceful, and ready to continue your journey. *Remember who you are.*

We all endure difficult times when we feel that we are completely alone. We feel disconnected and disempowered. We forget that although we have free will, there are specific lessons that we are incarnated to learn. Our souls manifest the circumstances that will help us to achieve this learning. The truth is, we are *never* alone. We can always ask the universe for help when we are not feeling in our power. The following meditation is designed to remind us that we can relax and go with the flow of what is manifested in our lives.

Meditation and Practice
Trust Your Spirit

1. Lie down on the floor with your spine straight. Close your eyes. Call your energy, your spirit, your thoughts into present time. Take deep, full, long breaths. With every breath you are breathing in brilliant, radiant, healing light. You are relaxing more and more with every breath you take. With every breath, you are releasing more and more tension. You are letting go. Soon there is no holding anywhere in your body. You are completely relaxed and supported by the floor.

2. Just as surely as your physical body is completely supported by the floor, your spirit is completely supported by the universe as you travel your path. Every person, every circumstance that enters your life is there by divine design in order to propel you onward and upward.

3. Let go of your judgment of every person and circumstance that enters your life. Dance with life and go gracefully with what is manifested for you, knowing that you are exactly where you're meant to be and that in every single moment, you are infinitely loved, supported, and guided.

Take a moment to relax into this truth. When you are ready, open your eyes. Go back into your day feeling safe and loved.

Chapter 21

CREATING YOUR REALITY

You can consciously create your reality, but you must draw your power into present time in order to do it. If your chi is stuck in the past or pushed forward into the future, you are not functioning with your full allotment of energy. Your energy powers the creation of your reality just as gasoline runs a car. If you are wasting gas by revisiting the past repeatedly, you are allowing yourself to use your fuel on the energy of fear. If you are using your energy to worry about the future—not *setting an intention* about your future, but worrying about what *might* be—again, you are wasting your energy on fear. This may well leave you unable to send out a strong intention to manifest what you desire with the energy of love *right now*. If the fuel that powers the creation of your reality is spread out into the past and future, there is not enough in this moment to bring into being the love-based reality you desire.

Forgiveness is the ultimate way of taking back your chi and is a powerful contributor to the process of manifesting your reality. We are empowered when we forgive those who have wronged us. When we forgive, it doesn't mean that we have to condone harmful behavior. It merely means that we let go of the anger and place appropriate boundaries with whoever has wronged us.

When we can't forgive, we are sending our chi back in time and attaching it to some person or event in the past. Remember that what you cannot forgive occurred for a reason. It carried a lesson for you that your spirit needed to learn. If you have not been able to forgive those in your past, not only are you left with less power in this moment, but, most importantly, *you have not learned the lesson you needed to learn.* Therefore, you can expect to be confronted by this *very same* lesson again, to give your soul another chance to learn it. This is an example of manifesting your reality unconsciously. When you can't forgive the past, you manifest the same situations in your present and your future life.

Remind yourself that the world is made of energy, and that energy follows thought and intention. When your core belief is fearful, assuming that "there is not enough," the energy of "not enough" will show up in your life.

The following are some of the many and varied points of view about the nature of creating your reality. Keep in mind that there are many different realities, and there are no right or wrong answers. Choose the viewpoint that works for you.

Neale Donald Walsch writes in *Conversations with God* that if you send out the energy of "I *want* a great job" or "I *wish* I had a boyfriend," you are creating the condition of *want* and *wish* in your life. You have the power to manifest your reality, but wanting something creates the condition of *want*. Just like your intentions, your manifestations can be based in either love or fear. If you let go of your sense of need, you can literally detach yourself from the energy of wanting, which is based in fear. Manifesting that arises from love will reflect your innermost self and reveal who you really are.

A journey of the soul has more to do with your *true nature* than what your mind perceives as your desires. By asking only for what you "want," you put limits on yourself. When you express an intention that is based in love and let go of fear-based neediness, you create the reality that is in alignment with your soul. Letting go of what you want, ironically, empowers you to realize your greatest potential.

Marianne Williamson writes in *A Return to Love* that if you communicate to the universe the thought of "What can I get?" you are sending out the vibration that your life is lacking. That thought will inevitably be reflected back to you through the circumstances of your life. When your intentions and actions manifest the spirit of "What can I give?" you are sending forth the conviction that you have more than enough. This thought, too, will be reflected back to you and take form in your life. It is the same with an attitude of gratitude and abundance. Walsch writes that the universe is one big Xerox machine that copies your thoughts. Florence Scovel Shinn asserts that along with affirmations that put your thoughts into words, you need to make a demonstration of your convictions. This is in alignment with Walsch, who says that we possess three levels of creative power: thought, word, and action. A thought is the first level of creation. From thought, you go to the second level, which is speaking words that spring from the "sponsoring thought." The third level is action out in the world.

You can say to yourself all day, "I am prosperous; I am abundant," but if your core belief is that you are not good enough, the universe registers that basic thought. Walsch acknowledges that it is very difficult to shift a core thought. Therefore, it is sometimes necessary to start the path of change by acting "as if," for example, acting as if you were already prosperous. This action alters your words, and that alteration eventually transforms your core belief.

Affirmations are a way to have an effect on the core thought that you wish to change. You may think and say a certain affirmation to yourself repeatedly, but if you don't act it out, you can stay stuck with the same core thought that you want to transform. Once you have identified the core thought that is based in fear, you can reclaim your chi with any of the Power Practices that work for you.

Go deep inside yourself and delve into what your core beliefs really are. When your basic beliefs are poverty and lack, your words and your actions will follow that theme. It is possible to change your core belief by looking at your life just as it is right now. Instead of seeing what you don't have, appreciate what you do have. Allow yourself to feel gratitude for all that is yours in this moment. This sets the stage for you to practice feeling abundant. Once you appreciate what you do have, you have opened the door to receive more, because your core belief becomes one of abundance.

As Caroline Myss says in her *Energy Anatomy* tapes, you may believe that you create your own reality, but if you blame anyone for anything that happened in your life, then you don't, at your core, truly believe it.

Some say it is not enough merely to have an abundant core thought. In John Gray's book *How to Get What You Want and Want What You Have,* he states that it is not enough simply to be grateful for the richness of your life. You must also set a strong intention for what you desire. In other words, not "I want," or "Please, please, please," but "I *know* that this will happen for me."

It's been said, too, that if you set the intention for something to occur in the future, then it *stays* in the future, where you never catch up to it. Norman Vincent Peale believed that you should be absolutely confident that something will happen for you, and be thankful for it, *right now.*

When Michelangelo created a sculpture, he believed it already existed within the stone. All he needed to do was expose it with his chisel and imagination. This is a metaphor for manifesting our futures. Theories of modern physics are in alignment with ancient philosophies in postulating that what we perceive as linear time is really a collective illusion. In "quantum reality," time does not "happen." It just *is.* If this is true, our futures or the many possible futures that are open to us are already in existence, just like the sculpture in the stone. In keeping with this concept, one technique for creating your reality is "to be your future self." Behave as though you already have everything you could ever desire. You are then inspired to *be* that person—joyful, abundant, and successful. The key in all of this is to create your reality in harmony with your soul, based in love, not fear. As Gary Zukav writes in *The Seat of the Soul,* "Gratifying needs that are based upon fear will not bring you to the touchstone of purpose. No matter how successful the personality becomes in accomplishing its goals, those goals will not be enough. Eventually it will hunger for the energy of its soul. Only when the personality begins to walk the path that its soul has chosen will it satisfy its hunger."

Let's incorporate all of these views into one practice and meditation:

Ten Steps for Creating Your Reality

1. Pull all of your energy into present time.

2. Using Spiritual Perspective, look at your life as a whole, projecting forward into your possible futures.

3. Appreciate all that is yours right now.

4. Recognize that you are exactly where you're meant to be.

5. Visualize what you want to manifest in your life.

6. Use your intuition to see whether what you want is based in love or fear.

7. Unplug your energy from any fear-based desires.

8. Let go of any neediness that is attached to this outcome.

9. Be grateful to the universe for the manifestation of what you want; appreciate that reality as if you already have it.

10. Be your future self now.

Meditation and Practice
Manifesting Your Future

1. Sit or lie in a comfortable position with your spine long and straight. Take deep, full, long breaths. Close your eyes. As you breathe, you are inhaling brilliant, clear, radiant, healing light. With every breath you take, the light enters all the cells in your body, dissolving the everyday cares and worries of this life as you remember what is really important. With every breath you take, you become more and more relaxed. Unplug your energy, your spirit, your thoughts from your past. Unplug with gratitude for the gifts and the lessons of the past, acknowledging that the past is what brought you to here and now. Unplug your energy, your spirit, your thoughts from your worries for the future. Remember that you are exactly where you're meant to be. Call your energy, your spirit, your thoughts into this moment. Feel the power of being fully present here and now.

2. Project your energy upward. Using your mind's eye, look down on your entire life. See your past to the left of your vision, your present directly below, and your future to the right. See your early years and the manifestation of the seeds that were planted there come to fruition in your present life.

3. Look at the beauty of your life in this moment. Acknowledge the love, the joy, the abundance that are yours right now, without anything having to change. Send up gratitude for the richness of your life as it is.

4. Recognize that you are exactly where you're meant to be.

5. See the seeds that have not yet come to fruition and those that you have just planted for your future life. Look into the future at what is possible for you and visualize your life unfolding exactly as you desire. Carry the image that all you desire is already there. It just needs to be uncovered. Now let your perspective return to your body, knowing that what you want already exists. Send up thanks for the beauty of your future life.

6. Be aware that your desires are love-based and joyful.

7. If you feel any fear or attachment, take this moment to pull your chi back to you.

8. Let go of any neediness or doubt or *wanting*. You don't need to *want* what is already yours.

9. Feel the full force of your joy and gratitude. Express this feeling to the universe.

10. Be your future self, the person who has already manifested everything that you want. Take a deep breath and open your eyes with confidence in your vision for the future.

A Final Note

It bears repeating that Chi Fitness consists of *practices*. Even when you know how to empower yourself, awareness and practice are required to put that knowledge to use in your daily life. When you give your power away through fear-based emotions, it is often very difficult to reclaim your chi, even if you understand the process and realize what you need to do. Not surprisingly, the more intense these emotions are, the more difficult it is to practice calling back and managing your energy. Don't be hard on yourself! We all need to experience our emotions, even the fear-based ones. It's an essential part of the process.

In the course of our lives, we often attach our energy to other people or outside events, believing that these individuals and occurrences define who we are. We look outside ourselves to prove our worth instead of realizing that our perfection, our power, lies within us. As you learn to stay in your power, you will need definition and validation from outside sources less and less. These practices are designed to empower you to deepen your connection to your authentic self, your perfection. You already possess all that you need.

Suggested Resources

Ageless Body, Timeless Mind by Deepak Chopra, M.D.

Anatomy of the Spirit by Caroline Myss, Ph.D.

Building Self-Esteem through Positive Discipline by Jane Nelson, Ed.D. (audiotape)

Conscious Breathing by Gay Hendricks, Ph.D.

Conversations with God by Neale Donald Walsch

Energy Anatomy by Caroline Myss, Ph.D. (audiotapes)

Energy Medicine by Donna Eden with David Feinstein

Hands of Light by Barbara Ann Brennan

How to Get What You Want and Want What You Have by John Gray

Many Lives, Many Masters by Brian L. Weiss, M.D.

The Philosophy of Soul and Matter by Gurudev Chitrabhanu

A Return to Love: Reflections on the Principles of <u>A Course in Miracles</u> by Marianne Williamson

The Seat of the Soul by Gary Zukav

Sound Body, Sound Mind by Andrew Weil, M.D.

Sounds of Healing by Mitchell L. Gaynor, M.D.

Spontaneous Healing by Andrew Weil, M.D.

Stalking the Wild Pendulum by Itzhak Bentov

The Tao of Physics by Fritjof Capra

Through Time into Healing by Brian L. Weiss, M.D.

Why People Don't Heal and How They Can by Caroline Myss, Ph.D.

The Writings of Florence Scovel Shinn by Florence Scovel Shinn

Acknowledgments

We have received inspiration from the works of many authors and teachers, especially Caroline Myss, Gary Zukav, Marianne Williamson, Neale Donald Walsch, Florence Scovel Shinn, and Moshe Feldenkrais. We also give our heartfelt thanks to Patricia van der Leun, Diane Reverand, and Janet Dery, for their guidance every step of the way, and to MaryEllen Hendricks, Yuki Hayasaki, Francine Langford, Andrew Brucker, and Richard Aquan, for their incomparable artistry, as well as Terry and Vasken Kalayjian, Lisa Knofla, Mark Romano, Jamie and Keith Styrcula, Luisa Tanno, Luisa Viladas, and Joyce Zimmerman, for their insights and encouragement. In addition, we'd like to thank all of our wonderful clients and instructors at Chi Fitness, in particular those who participated in the focus groups for this book.

Visit www.chifitness.com for more information.

Index

About the Authors

SUE BENTON is the founder and President of Chi Fitness. Sue has been exploring movement forms throughout her life. She created the core Chi Fitness classes, including Chi Dance, Chi Sculpt, and Dance Workout. Sue has been teaching for fourteen years and also directs the teacher training program at Chi Fitness. She is a graduate of Chatham College and received her master's degree in public administration from the University of Pittsburgh. Sue lives with her husband, Drew Denbaum, and her two children, Andy and Ali, in Westport, Connecticut.

DREW DENBAUM is the Managing Director of Chi Fitness. A graduate of Yale University, he is also an award-winning writer, director, and actor in film, television, and the theater. Drew is the father of two children, Evan and Daria. He has practiced Jain Meditation for over twenty-five years.